Trauma in Otolaryngology

Jayita Das

Trauma in Otolaryngology

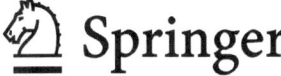 Springer

Jayita Das
Department of Otolaryngology
Pondicherry Institute of Medical Science
Kalapet
Pondicherry
India

ISBN 978-981-10-6360-2   ISBN 978-981-10-6361-9   (eBook)
https://doi.org/10.1007/978-981-10-6361-9

Library of Congress Control Number: 2017958869

Printed on acid-free paper

This Springer imprint is published by Springer Nature
The registered company is Springer Nature Singapore Pte Ltd.
The registered company address is: 152 Beach Road, #21-01/04 Gateway East, Singapore 189721, Singapore

Foreword

Trauma in ENT practice is fairly common, but its severity varies from trivial to a life-threatening emergency such as airway obstruction. The general practitioner is taught the basics of treating minor trauma and the initial lifesaving skills in dealing with major trauma before transferring the patient/casualty to the appropriate center for specialized care. The ENT surgeon, on the other hand, is expected to manage any ENT emergency regardless of whether he or she is practicing in a standalone clinic or a tertiary referral hospital. However, the emergency surgical skills are not learned fully during the training phase, due to many reasons, one being paucity of time and the second being exposure to real emergencies.

This practical textbook written by Dr Jayita Das—associate professor, Department of ENT, Head & Neck Surgery, Pondicherry Institute of Medical Sciences—gives a detailed description of all kinds of trauma that an ENT or casualty medical officer may have to face. The pathophysiology, management principles, techniques, as well as prognosis have been described along with function restoration. I compliment the author for taking up a topic which is applicable and useful, for both a GP and the ENT doctor. The topics have been dealt with systematically and covered in depth with good illustrations. The quiz at the end attempts to test the reader in assessing his/her level of competence after reading this excellent book. This book is recommended for all medical practitioners and especially ENT doctors. I congratulate the author for her excellent overview of the subject and clarity in expression. I wish her the very best for the success of this maiden attempt and wish her more success in future publications.

A. Ravikumar, MS, DNB, DLORCS (England), FAMS,
Department of ENT, Head & Neck Surgery,
Sri Ramachandra Medical College & Research Institute,
Chennai, India

Preface

If only the human body could handle trauma as well as biotechnology stocks do.

Spy novelist Alex Berenson was perhaps ignorant of the truth about the human body, and its ability to handle trauma, better and more efficiently than one could imagine.

But there is a caveat here. It does matter which part of the human body suffers the trauma and what is the magnitude of the injury.

Trauma can range from major to miniscule, physical to psychological, and emotional to electrical. Major trauma to the major organ systems—the cranial cavity, airway, chest and lungs, abdomen, and pelvis and long bones—is usually fatal or at least accompanied by a very high level of morbidity. Minor trauma, on the other hand, may often go unnoticed and unremembered. Physical trauma may be externally obvious, but psychological trauma may fester for long periods of time and do even more serious damage to the sufferer. Emotional trauma could stop the heart in its tracks, literally, as could an electric shock running through the body.

It now becomes clear that it is almost impossible to predict or preempt trauma and, further still, to formulate treatment policies that might apply to trauma in general. Each type of trauma, and the body part it affects, must be considered as a separate entity, and suitable management protocols devised.

Most of the literature on trauma describes the issues or problems surrounding the wound and perhaps some host factors such as health, nutritional status, and immunity. It would therefore be interesting to look at how numerous other factors, mainly social and economic, directly or indirectly impact the outcomes arising out of trauma or its treatment.

For example, much trauma or injurious insult results from urbanization of societies and the occurrence of motor vehicle accidents. Also, increased life spans, artificial life support, and assisted reproduction have added their peculiar imprint upon the evolution of trauma in many parts of the globe. All these, coupled with the monetary and educational standards of the population, and the health infrastructure of that region, play an important role. They also define how a particular kind of trauma might be dealt with using a particular level of expertise and thereby the final consequence of the particular event.

There are some unique characteristics of trauma in ENT practice. Spanning the entire gamut of major and minor trauma, there are also factors which should take into consideration demographic profiles and medicolegal aspects, besides the actual business of management of the said trauma. For example, variations among different age groups, rural and urban populations, and healthcare facilities available could impact the way trauma is treated. Outcomes would also vary accordingly. It is imperative to follow sound clinical practices, evidence-based medicine, and, of course, a gut instinct in order to ensure that the best outcomes result from the treatment of trauma.

Because trauma is sudden and unpredictable, the outcomes of managing it have a telling impact upon the quality of life of the patient and reflect on the quality of healthcare facility in general and the doctor in particular. This book therefore endeavors to remind all practitioners of ENT the core principles of management of trauma in this specialty. The chapters describing trauma in each region in the head and neck are presented in a simple and comprehensive manner, with a background or introduction about the relevant anatomy and pathophysiology, the body or main text dealing with the clinical implications, and finally rounding off with a section on prognosis, best practice, future directions, and/or practical applications. A brief and gentle reminder of the embryological development of the ear and nose would hopefully serve to sensitize the reader to the implications of trauma to these organs of special sense. The book follows an easy storytelling style instead of a bullet-point handbook format, specifically with the aim to suit the casual reader, slow reader, methodical reader, or even the reader who has no time to read!

The first three chapters deal with the history of trauma care and general principles in trauma, while the next three specifically discuss trauma in the ear, nose, and throat regions. Chapter 7 describes eye trauma in the context of the ENT surgeon, while Chap. 8 is devoted to foreign bodies, which may be considered to form a particular type of trauma or external insult. Controversies regarding trauma in various regions of the head and neck are discussed in the respective chapters. Chapter 9 challenges trainees and practitioners alike with case scenarios taken from both institutional and independent settings. The last section provides a quick review in the form of a quiz.

It is hoped that this book shall be able to provide everything the ENT practitioner wanted to know about trauma in this specialty and that the management of trauma will turn out to be a gratifying experience for both patient and doctor, in spite of the daunting implications it carries for most individuals.

Kalapet, Pondicherry, India   Jayita Das

Acknowledgment

The author wishes to convey her heartfelt gratitude to the following:

Professor Ravikumar—mentor and role model—for writing the Foreword of this book.

Patients, resident doctors, peers, and superiors at the Pondicherry Institute of Medical Sciences for the opportunity and purpose to take up this enterprise.

My colleagues in the Department of Radiology—Dr Linu Kuruvilla and Dr Sreshtha Hegde—have helped me immensely with the sourcing of the images. A special word of thanks goes to my residents Paresh Pramod Naik and Roshan Marie Thomas for being friends, critics, and sounding boards.

And my family without whose love, patience, and support this would not have been possible.

Photo credits for the images of outer ear trauma also go to Dr Paresh Naik.

Springer publishers for the valuable guidance and encouragement.

About the Author

Jayita Das is an ENT specialist with more than 20 years of operative experience in all areas of general otolaryngology practice, in both the private sector and institutional settings dealing with postgraduate training. She is a firm believer in the philosophy of patient-centered, evidence-based practice and an active educator at both the undergraduate and postgraduate levels.

Her published works include more than 15 articles in indexed journals, in addition to textbook chapters in the Medscape (eMedicine) Online References. She is a reviewer/editorial board member for several indexed national and international journals. She authored the book *Optimizing Medicine Residency Training Programs*, published by IGI Global in October 2015, and contributed a chapter on medical errors in another publication by IGI Global.

She is also an avid mother, homemaker, trekker, travel writer, photographer and amateur musician, and is currently engaged in academic practice at a tertiary care facility in Pondicherry.

Contents

Part: I

Principles of Trauma Management in ENT, Head and Neck

Introduction and Historical Backdrop

Learning Objectives
- To learn the basis of trauma management from a historical perspective
- To study how the management has evolved over the years with improved outcomes
- To understand what challenges remain in the optimal management of trauma

1.1 The Background Is the Battleground

The word trauma is derived from an alteration of "troma" for the Greek word "titroskein" (to wound) or "tetrainein" (to pierce) and is believed to have been first used around the year 1693.

As may be expected, accounts of trauma and its treatment date back to ancient times—almost as long ago as 10,000 BC—when human civilization developed and territorial wars were waged between persons and communities. Historical accounts have been found in Mesopotamia, Egypt, Greece, Rome, China, India, Austria, and Germany and include descriptions of craniotomies and trephinations being done to evacuate hematomas. These offer interesting insights into the understanding of the human body and its ability to handle trauma. The Egyptian and Greco-Roman times witnessed large-scale battles and a gradual transition to the management of war wounds and war casualties. The Romans almost perfected this stratagem and established "valetudinaria" [1] all across their lands in which the victims and survivors of wars could be attended to expeditiously and methodically. In ancient India under the rule of Ashoka, casualties of war were attended to expertly with the help of indigenously designed ambulances, skilled surgeons, and a support system provided by the womenfolk who cooked and cared for the wounded soldiers—probably the first evidence of a nursing service!

© Springer Nature Singapore Pte Ltd. 2018
J. Das, *Trauma in Otolaryngology*, https://doi.org/10.1007/978-981-10-6361-9_1

The rise of science and medicine during the Renaissance paved the way for a scientific approach to injury, but many more lessons were yet to be learnt. For one, hypovolemic shock due to hemorrhage was not understood though it was being treated with ephedrine-like substances derived from medicinal plants. The first breakthrough came with the French scientist Ambrose Pare in the sixteenth century, who propounded techniques such as ligation, effective treatment of gunshot injuries, attention to diet and nutrition to aid recovery, and the use of artificial limbs for those undergoing amputation.

Napoleon's general Dominique Larrey took this even further with the need for speedy evacuation and evaluation of soldiers in battle, making the most of the immediate post-injury period where the survivor was still stunned out enough to withstand an operative procedure without the help of anesthesia. He also provided great insights into the organization of military evacuations and strategies for the same at various possible targets of the enemy forces.

It is thus seen that the management of trauma emerged from the warfront and the military and then made its way to the civil urban setting, though medical milestones such as the introduction of aseptic techniques, antiseptics, and antibiotics made a significant contribution to improving the outcomes. During the First World War, the average time for evacuation was 12–18 h, with tamponade, splinting, and debridement the main modes of management, and it is therefore understandable that there was a high price to pay. Most of the soldiers did not make it beyond the battlefront and those who did were maimed for life.

A dramatic shift was seen during the Second World War with the arrival of evacuation by air, and the time for transportation was cut down by half. Blood loss and shock were avoided to a large extent, and patients were brought to a proper hospital where adequate care and treatment could be provided. The mortality rate was reduced, but morbidity was still very high, and things did not progress much beyond the acute care of trauma. Surgery and rehabilitation were still to be developed. Subsequent great wars further refined strategy till not only acute management of trauma but also dealing with its aftermath—rehabilitation—became watchwords in trauma care.

1.2 The Battleground in the Backyard

Urbanization, industrialization, and motorization of society eventually shifted the gears of trauma care toward civilian life but here too with the same principles as in the military, namely, evacuation, acute care, and definitive management, in that order. Roughly at the same time in both Europe and North America, namely, the late 1960s and early 1970s, dedicated hospitals for the wounded and injured were set up and came to be known as trauma centers. In April 1969, the first trauma center was established in Baltimore, Maryland, USA.

Treatment protocols for trauma soon followed and in 1976 the American College of Surgeons Committee on Trauma (ACSCOT) published the first "Optimal Criteria" report, which formed the basis of the ATLS (Advanced Trauma Life Support) guidelines that are known so well today. Trauma registries were also started by the same professional body as above and were effectively used for the establishment of verified and validated trauma centers that met all the requirements mandated by law and public policy. Five dedicated trauma centers were established in North America by 1995 [2].

The impact or trauma on civilian life is so pervasive in the modern world that several other dimensions have been added to trauma management. The chief among these is prevention and governmental regulation. It is easily understood that here, more than anywhere else, much can be gained from simple preventive strategies. Traffic rules and regulations, law and order, car and automobile manufacturing and design, and public awareness and education pay very rich dividends.

Prehospital care is the second aspect. The availability and infrastructure of ambulance services, communications technology to facilitate rapid and timely evacuation, well-trained paramedical staff and the principles of triage, and the resources to transfer to designated centers for trauma care are all involved in this.

In most countries, health provisions are a governmental priority, and in the West, even trauma is included in this. During times of conflict and strife, economic resources are naturally pressed into extending trauma services to the defense forces. At peacetime, however, the same commitment may be missing from the provision of trauma care to the civilian population. In North America too, federal funding initially given for the establishment of well-known trauma centers eventually shrunk to such levels that many of these hospitals were forced to down their shutters or downgrade to general or even acute care hospitals but not wholly dedicated to covering trauma.

1.3   The Daily Battle

Treatment philosophies and physician demographics further added to the deepening crisis as far as trauma services were concerned. Damage control surgery or a conservative approach to trauma means that while acute care is provided to trauma survivors in the intensive care setting, more time is spent in the hospital and various diagnostic steps, while the actual surgical management of trauma takes second place. Younger, dynamic general surgeons with an interest in trauma are thus not attracted toward this highly demanding but fulfilling career. Even subspecialty training in acute care surgery deals mainly with surgical emergencies and not exclusively with trauma, which really deserves a place of its own. As a result of this, other subspecialists such as plastic, cardiothoracic vascular, maxillofacial, orthopedic, neurosurgery, and of late ENT are involved in providing services jointly, leading to confusion and chaos in many hospitals. Particularly disturbing is the fact that different subspecialists expect and demand differential wages or reimbursement as the primary physicians of trauma care. For example, neurosurgeons are not only in short supply compared to general surgeons but also possess a level of expertise that commands better remuneration. Having them as frontline providers of trauma services could be a major economic drain on resources. At the same time, head injury is the first and foremost problem to be dealt with in trauma management, and so a neurosurgeon is eminently suitable to be the trauma surgeon of first contact on a call day.

The paradox is evident—a less qualified or competent general surgeon versus a costly but expert trauma care provider—thus making the delivery of trauma services that much more challenging. Training of emergency trauma surgeons falls pitifully short of making a consummate trauma care provider who can single-handedly manage a case of complex trauma at least as far as decision making is concerned. This is important to understand because even though various specialists may be involved in the trauma team, there is usually one leader or person of authority who has the primary responsibility and is in a position to make important decisions in the provision of care to the trauma patient.

The growing participation of women in the medical—and surgical—specialties has also caused significant changes. While striving to balance family and career, women graduate as doctors, and even surgeons, but stay away from trauma. Though lifestyle issues are a concern with male surgeons too, it is by far greater in the case of women. Working in shifts and protected time during the training period could be useful and is indeed the norm in many institutions. This could indeed work well as long as there is a continuum of care, which again might be a point of concern in some places with poorer infrastructure and staffing.

While this may sound very straightforward and simplistic, it is not difficult to pick out the inherent challenges in trauma management, which, more often than not, has repercussions well beyond the boundaries of individual persons and diseases. The very fact that designated trauma centers are the way to go to deliver effective care to trauma patients means infrastructure, staffing, morale, and culture—things which almost overwhelm the scientific approach when considered alone. Trauma specialists have a hectic lifestyle with intense and irregular work schedules, often having to provide services at nearby or sister institutions. Such dynamics naturally mean that older (and more experienced) staff gradually shy away from providing trauma services even as they stay actively involved in other forms of acute and emergency surgical care, as accepted by most hospitals and institutions.

The insurance coverage of trauma is a more worrying trend, one that is proving to be a disincentive for its actual provision. As trauma care services typically use up great resources of manpower and material, insurers are chary of providing cover for the same, even though accident and injury coverage is widespread and sometimes even cost-effective for the individual because an accident is after all a matter of chance, and paying a small premium to cover such a remote risk is well worth it. One clever but unfortunate way that insurance companies maximize on their profit margins is to give the impression that a matter of chance is simply that—a freak incident—and thereby does not deserve the investment that automatically goes into it if it were to actually occur. They therefore discourage medical professionals from providing emergency services by proffering concessions on their annual premiums if they desist from such activities. Little is it realized that such practices put a huge stress on existing resources thereby leading to suboptimal outcomes for trauma in many places.

Smaller, less equipped, and sparsely staffed trauma centers are often reluctant or unable to provide services beyond first aid and readily refer to higher centers without a proper evaluation of the situation. Many a time, the patient might not even require further referrals, but doctors would always want to be on the safer side and therefore often second guess themselves as to the optimum management of a trauma patient. The risk of malpractice litigation is also disproportionately high, thereby leading to a commensurate decrease in the enthusiasm for trauma practice.

Public perception and governmental regulation play major roles in providing trauma services, the impact of which is noteworthy. In North America, trauma systems have emerged which take into account how a trauma center should be classified, the availability and access to communications technology that ensures rapid evacuation for the victims, the manufacturing and design of ambulances which are not only well equipped but also able to safely transfer patients from the scene of accident to the trauma center, the staffing and training of medical professionals dealing with trauma, and the meticulous maintenance of trauma registries and data that could be used in the evaluation of trauma services and further shape public policy. Based on the above criteria, trauma centers can be initially categorized into four levels—the area emergency hospitals are the first and highest level of services and are fully equipped as far as infrastructure, staffing, and other resources are concerned. The general emergency service hospital is the next level where a less intense environment of trauma care exists, and referral to a higher center might be carried out. The community trauma center has just the basic facilities to provide first aid and resuscitation, and the rest are uncategorized because they lack even this. Five thrust areas are recognized—government regulation and policy, infrastructure, training, communication, and active service—and the three crucial steps in order to achieve the above are to recognize the need, to implement appropriate orders or action, and to audit the results.

Funding for such trauma centers has been erratic, thus leading to closure or downgrading of many first-level trauma centers. As trauma and emergency services are more often than not provided free of cost, a lack of funding would lead to the natural decline in services. Insurers and third party payers further aggravate the situation by giving incentives for containment of costs. This might well mean that the full range of services is not provided to the trauma patient.

Patients also like to seek treatment at hospitals of their choice and thus seek emergency or first aid alone at even fully equipped trauma centers. As the law mandates compulsory provision of first aid irrespective of the patient's ability to pay, many hospitals end up providing free services and then not being compensated for having done so if the patient decides to seek definitive treatment elsewhere. This then acts as a deterrent for providing trauma care in the first place, and many institutions that are otherwise reputed may not be involved in trauma care services at all. On the other hand, if a hospital can competently handle trauma, it can also continue to grow on the basis of this, and eventually other services are also improved, thereby leading to overall cost-effectiveness in the long run.

1.4   The Battle Begins

ENT or otolaryngology specialists were previously not a traditional component of trauma teams in military deployment; they were first officially recruited in Iraq by American forces seeking to free the country from the despotic ruler Saddam Hussein. Along with neurosurgeons, oral and maxillofacial surgeons, and ophthalmic specialists, otolaryngologists too formed an important part of the multispecialty head and neck trauma services team [3]. This makes eminent sense because otolaryngologists are intimately familiar with head and neck anatomy as a whole, and a good number are also specifically trained in head and neck oncology, reconstruction, and rehabilitation, thereby rendering them highly proficient in the management of complex trauma of this region.

The head and neck form not just a distinctive region of the human body but also comprise of a multitude of tissue types and organs with specific characteristics. There is the brain in the cranial cavity which is connected to a network of nerves and pathways that control and move the human being. There are blood vessels so tiny that they are almost invisible, and others so large and spread out that they pose a monumental challenge to the control of hemorrhage in case of injury. There are organs of the special senses, which, if damaged, seriously affect the quality of life even if the extent of injury is minor. All such injuries to the special sense organs are therefore considered grievous. Last but not least, the muscles, bones, and soft tissues of this region have remarkable properties and could significantly alter the external appearance of a person in the event of trauma and its aftermath. Esthetics and social acceptability are therefore important issues when dealing with trauma in the head and neck region.

The head and neck are also common ground for a plethora of specialist doctors. Neurosurgeons, plastic surgeons, dentists and maxillofacial surgeons, ophthalmologists, and otorhinolaryngologists all vie for space in this small, compact portion of human anatomy. Many a time, all must work together or in tandem, and it goes without saying that often each one of these specialists must have an innate or explicit understanding of each other's territory and surgical domain and healthy respect for each other's expertise.

Trauma in the head and neck must be evaluated and treated according to standard trauma protocols, and not in an isolated manner. While dealing with trauma, it is imperative to have a basis for deciding what comes first, in other words, the order in which one region might take precedence over another in terms of urgency and gravity of the situation.

For most practitioners of ENT (otorhinolaryngology)—be it in an institutional or independent setting—trauma is either a vague concept and occasional occurrence or a matter of daily work. Given the nature of highly specialized and compartmentalized practice in ENT, major trauma would most certainly be encountered as a byproduct of tertiary care practice as a part of multidisciplinary management. At the other extreme, minor trauma involving the ear, nose, throat, head, or neck could plague a physician of first contact or a primary care practitioner.

1.5   The Rules of the Battle

1.5.1   Diagnosis

Diagnosis begins with the hierarchy of suspicion, which, in other words, is in the following order:

1. Common presentation of common diseases must be considered first.
2. Uncommon presentation of common diseases can be considered next.
3. Common presentation of rare disease is next in line.
4. Uncommon presentation of rare disease is to be considered last.

In trauma, this method of thinking may not always be necessary but could be useful when the patient is not in a condition to provide the history or in the presence of pre-existing disease or medical conditions and in instances of foul play.

1.5.2   Classification and Types of Trauma

Trauma can be broadly classified into two types—penetrating and non-penetrating. The latter may be further grouped into the following categories—blunt trauma, thermal or chemical injury, crush and avulsion injuries, barotraumas, and blast overpressure. Blunt trauma may cause injury by several mechanisms such as stretch and shear, torsion or rotation, and acceleration or deceleration.

There are many other ways in which trauma could be classified (Table 1.1).

Depending on severity and presence or absence of polytrauma and comorbidities:

1. Major/complicated
2. Minor/simple

Depending primarily on the condition of the wound and the presence or absence of debris:

1. Clean
2. Contaminated

Depending on external factors only or that caused by medical intervention:

1. Environmental
2. Iatrogenic

Table 1.1 Classification of trauma

Penetrating	Clean	Major	Environmental
Non-penetrating	Contaminated	Minor	Iatrogenic

Indeed, it is plain to see that these classifications exist and are important mainly because:

1. They indicate the level and scope of intervention required.
2. They serve as prognostic factors and determine outcome.
3. They may be used to explore the harmful effects, side effects, or complications of a medical or surgical procedure. In other words, they provide a database for the investigation of medical errors.

Classification aside, dealing with trauma requires a common sense approach, in addition to scientific methods and principles. It is also important to remember that given the emergent nature of the majority of cases of trauma, it is not often the medical professional who is called upon to deal with the sufferer but a layman. This means that the patient, family member or friend, or simply a bystander among the general public might be the first person to intervene.

This might or might not include first aid, application of harmful substances with the belief of providing relief but which might actually make the problem worse, the time lag between the trauma and the arrival of patient to a medical facility, the interval between arrival and therapeutic intervention, and finally the time required for return to normalcy or functional ability.

All the above factors are crucial in determining the final outcome of an episode of trauma.

1.6   Winning the Battle

As in any disease, everything starts with a diagnosis. History of symptoms, a meticulous examination, and a solid theoretical knowledge base and cognitive recall pave the way for sound clinical analysis and judgment—the two strengths that are necessary for the execution of successful treatment. So it is with the correct and precise diagnosis that one can hope to carry out the optimum management of any illness. Nowhere is this more important than in trauma and, even more so, trauma encountered by an ENT specialist.

As is common in many modern healthcare settings, most ailments are managed in a multidisciplinary setting. Roles are carefully carved out (pun intended!) for the specialties that might be involved in managing trauma. The neurosurgeon, general surgeon, otolaryngologist, ophthalmologist, and plastic surgeon may be directly or indirectly involved in each other's domain. The orthopedist may also be an important component in this process depending on the nature and extent of the trauma.

It is therefore imperative that while making a diagnosis, it is the patient one must have in mind instead of the specialty. For example, a nosebleed in an unconscious patient is not just a case of "epistaxis" but actually a "head injury with fracture(s) of the facial skeleton with epistaxis [with or without polytrauma]." The implications would differ hugely give or take any one of the components of such a diagnosis.

Conclusion

The history of trauma management reveals interesting facts about the crucial factors responsible for good outcomes—sound policy, good communication, and solid infrastructure—to name a few. In tandem with scientific and technological progress, it is these factors that are the final determinants in minimizing morbidity arising from trauma.

References

1. Trunkey DD. The emerging crisis in trauma care: a history and definition of the problem. Clin Neurosurg. 2007;54:200–5
2. Bazzoli GJ, Madiera KJ, Cooper GF, McKenzie EJ, Maier RV. Progress in the development of trauma systems in the United States: results of a national survey. JAMA. 1995;273:395–401
3. Brennan J. Experience of first deployed otolaryngology team in Operation Iraqi Freedom: the changing face of combat injuries. Otolaryngol Head Neck Surg. 2006;134(1):100–5

Learning Objectives
- To understand the basic principles and protocols in trauma management
- To learn about the supportive treatments and their relevance in managing trauma
- To consider the medicolegal aspects of trauma management and their practical applications

2.1   General Principles

Optimal management of trauma, as with any other type of disorder or disease, starts with the basics. On the one hand, these basics involve rapid control of the situation physically to ensure survival of the trauma victim, and this is done as per the ATLS guidelines. On the other hand, the basics involve going to the background in which the trauma or injury has occurred or, in other words, doing a root cause analysis (RCA) of the situation. The RCA must take into account the following.

2.1.1   Time of Injury

Specifically how much time has elapsed following the injury and whether the "golden hour" (the first 1 h) is applicable.

The golden hour concept was introduced by R. Adams Cowley in the 1960s and referred to the critical time period after trauma during which the patient should have received medical attention in order to avoid a fatality. This has now given way to the concept of the "platinum minutes" or the "Platinum Ten" which underscores the need for immediate medical attention for a trauma victim in order to reduce

morbidity and improve outcomes. The platinum 10 min refer to the first 10 min following injury and may be subdivided as the first 1 min for primary survey, the next
5 min for stabilizing and resuscitating the patient, and the last 4 min for transportation to the nearest medical or trauma center.

2.1.2 Place of Injury

The scene of injury, whether domestic or public. Domestic injuries include accidental falls or collisions, gas explosions or leaks, electrical short circuits causing burns
or shocks, inhalation or ingestion of foreign bodies leading to impaction and airway
obstruction, suicidal injuries such as attempted hanging or cut-throat, or homicidal
attacks and child, spousal, or elder abuse.

2.1.3 Nature of Injury

Ruling out the presence of impacted foreign bodies; contamination with noxious
substances such as gases, fumes, or chemicals; and implicating weapons or sharp
objects where strangulation, gunshot, or knife injuries are suspected. Special cases
such as drowning or asphyxia may mechanically compromise the airway in addition
to the damage caused by hypoxia or hypothermia. Postural drainage for clearing the
airway of aspirated substances and manual evacuation of the airway must be quickly
instituted. Incriminating or precipitating factors such as alcohol intoxication,
administration of poisons, or coexisting metabolic or systemic disease must be
looked into as possible causes and risk factors.

The history taking must include the details of previous intervention if any, especially administration of medications and fluids, pre-injury photographs if available,
and accounts of passersby or rescuers if such details cannot be provided by the
patient.

2.1.4 Coverage of Costs

Provision of lifesaving first aid is a legal obligation of all healthcare
establishments and is usually carried out without consideration of costs involved
in a professional, ethical, and impartial manner. But wide variations may be
seen across the globe as to the extent and quality of such care. Sooner or later,
the issue of expenditure involved in the management of the trauma survivor
becomes crucial, and just as in the acute control of the situation, a rapid and
efficient decision making process must ensure the continuum of care and take it
to its logical end. Different teams working together add to this problem, and the
legal and financial elements of trauma care, with or without insurance coverage,
need to be worked out in an expedient manner to minimize hassles for the victim
and family.

2.1.5 Rehabilitation

This varies greatly from case to case and is discussed in relation to the relevant trauma. In this regard too, the pre-injury status of the patient, occupation, social and demographic profile, psychological status, level of handicap if any, involvement of the family or caregivers, financial solvency, and so on play major roles in the final outcome. A consideration of the same must be in the background of even the acute and early management of the patient in order to ensure seamless integration into the management process.

2.1.6 In Cases of Polytrauma

In cases of polytrauma, the principles of management are the following.

2.1.6.1 Triage

This is the process of sorting of patients who have suffered trauma and applies to the acute care setting especially in cases of mass casualties. It is based on a system of color coding and indicates the time required to transfer the patient to definitive care and is as follows:

Black—deceased (no further treatment required; arrange for proper disposal of the body)

Red—emergent/immediate (within 10 min)

Amber—urgent (within 60 min)

Yellow—expedient (within 120 min)

Green—minor (within 240 min)

Blue—discharged (advice to review at a later date, or periodically and as needed, may be given)

The amount of blood loss must be assessed as accurately as possible because this determines the prognosis of the acute care management of the patient. Loss of 100% of total blood volume in 1 h is invariably fatal, while the loss of 50% or more of total blood volume in the first 4 h means that the patient is in a critical condition and expedient management is called for, and the loss of more than 150 ml of blood in an hour is considered severe and implies close monitoring and vigilance for the onset of complications. The combination of hypothermia, that is, a core body temperature of 35 °C or less, with death occurring at 32 °C (not compatible with survival); acidosis (pH 7.2 or less); and coagulopathy indicated by an international normalized ratio (INR) of 1.5 or more, is known as the lethal triad because it is the harbinger of fatal complications.

2.1.6.2 The Airway

The airway must be maintained in the following ways in order of increasing sophistication:

1. Spontaneous on room air or oxygenation by nasal catheter
2. Bag-mask ventilation

3. Laryngoscopy and endotracheal intubation
4. Awake fiber optic intubation
5. Nasotracheal intubation
6. Intubation with bougie
7. Laryngeal mask airway
8. Video-assisted laryngoscopy
9. Cricothyroidotomy
10. Tracheotomy (open surgical or percutaneous dilatational procedure)

2.1.6.3 Imaging

Imaging is one of the crucial requirements in acute trauma care, and in the case of polytrauma, it typically involves plain X-rays of the thorax, abdomen, pelvis, and long limbs, focused abdominal ultrasound for trauma (FAST) or a vascular Doppler, multidetector computerized tomography (MDCT), and magnetic resonance imaging (MRI) to rule out diffuse axonal injury or spinal cord injuries.

X-rays may be taken for bony injuries of the facial skeleton, but with the advent of CT scanning, especially 3D CT, X-rays have become redundant. For suspected foreign bodies in the oropharynx, X-rays may not be helpful as there is overshadow from the bony structures of the mandible.

Two modalities are available in CT scanning—the fan beam CT and the cone beam CT [1]. The latter is considered superior as it delivers less radiation doses and the long-term side effects of radiation exposure such as the risk of developing malignancy, infertility, liver dysfunction, and lung fibrosis. It is worthwhile keeping in mind that the radiation exposure to the patient from HRCT temporal bone is 2.5–3.5 mSv (the equivalent of 25–30 chest X-rays) and the exposure to the lens of the eye is the maximum (1.5–2.0 mSv or 15–20 X-rays).

Given the volume of use of CT scan in trauma management, most centers dealing with trauma are able to realize their return on investment (ROI) in as quickly as 7 months of use [2]. Laboratory tests are done as per the requirements of the individual patients.

In addition, when unexplained hemorrhage occurs or is suspected, interventional radiology may be undertaken and includes angiography, transarterial embolization (TAE), and the use of fibrin glue and zeolites through emergency endoscopic procedures.

2.1.6.4 Multidisciplinary Team

Orthopedic injuries in the setting of polytrauma may complicate the situation gravely because of the risk of fat embolism, which may occur with the collection of 150 ml liquid fat in trauma involving the long limbs. Pelvic crush injuries may result in disseminated intravascular coagulation (DIC) and acute renal shutdown. Vascular compromise and gangrene may start to set in and would necessitate urgent debridement, fasciotomy, or amputation, in that order. Venous thromboembolism, subacute inflammatory response system (SIRS), and counteracting anti-inflammatory response system (CARS) are other sentinel events that determine the prognosis. Both SIRS and CARS determine prognosis in the first week of trauma; therefore, current guidelines recommend that any orthopedic intervention be limited to limb stabilization, and not definitive fixation or surgical intervention, or what is better known as damage control surgery.

Neurosurgical concerns may sometimes be in contravention to the management principles of trauma in other parts of the body, and close cooperation and coordination among surgical teams is paramount. As head injury must be optimally treated as a first measure, certain anomalies may first be apparent to the trauma team but nevertheless respected. These include the avoidance of a nasogastric tube (to minimize the risk of meningitis), avoidance of mannitol (as its effect on reducing brain edema is controversial), avoidance of steroids (as these are believed to lower the threshold for seizures), avoidance of hypotonic fluids or crystalloids (as these might increase intracranial pressure), and the use of prophylactic anticonvulsants (as the potential for post head injury seizures is high, especially in vulnerable populations such alcoholics and epileptics). The use of prophylactic antibiotics is disputed in the absence of contamination of other body tissues. An important thing is to avoid secondary insults such as hypoxia, hypotension, hypocarbia, hypercapnia, hyperglycemia, hyperthermia, hypothermia, acidosis, and coagulopathy, the last three forming the lethal triad that can precipitously worsen the prognosis of the patient.

2.2 Management Protocol

The advanced trauma life support (ATLS) is a standard protocol for the management of trauma and consists of the following components that should be executed in a stepwise manner:

1. *The primary survey* is done in order to assess the acute condition that might prove fatal to the patient, for example, an assessment that rapid and exsanguinating hemorrhage is taking place, or that the patient is asphyxiating because of an airway obstruction.
2. *The second step is resuscitation* or the immediate control of the cause that might prove fatal or terminal—in the above example, it would be control of the bleeding with tamponade or tourniquet and an emergency tracheotomy, along with rapid infusion of fluids to contain the hypovolemia and ventilator assistance, respectively.
3. A *secondary survey* must follow in order to systematically assess and identify any other injuries present.
4. *Definitive care* is then planned in a methodical manner taking into consideration the current scenario and best practice principles, and the comprehensive management of the patient is evolved.

In many cases, the primary survey and resuscitation must be carried out simultaneously or concurrently and may merge into each other in a single step.

The components of the primary survey include the airway with control of the cervical spine, attention to breathing and ventilation, maintenance of the circulation with control of hemorrhage, managing any dysfunction of the central nervous system, and control and evaluation of exposure to noxious stimuli in a controlled environment. A mini-neurological examination may be carried out at the prehospital stage to look for alertness, response to verbal commands, response to pain, and size and reaction of the pupils. Immediate life-threatening conditions in the thoracic compartment, for example, airway obstruction, tension pneumothorax, massive hemothorax (more than 1500 ml blood in a hemithorax), open pneumothorax ("sucking wound"), flail segment with pulmonary contusion, and cardiac tamponade (that is almost always due to a penetrating injury), must be addressed immediately.

Trauma protocols usually revolve around the four cardinal principles of rapid primary survey, resuscitation, detailed secondary survey, and reevaluation, as described above, with attention being focused on what is better known as the ABCDE of acute trauma care:

A—airway,
B—breathing (ventilation)
C—circulation
D—disability/neurological deficit
E—exposure or environmental threat

Of late, the ATLS protocol has been modified to CABDE, emphasizing the urgency of ensuring circulation as the starting point of trauma management. This is also the protocol in any sort of circulatory collapse as in the case of acute myocardial infarction. In practical terms, this means that cardiac massage or resuscitation must take precedence over the establishment of a patent airway, though in the majority of instances, both of these must be executed simultaneously or closely in tandem, beginning with restoring the circulation. In case of trauma, there may be massive exsanguination and/or cardiogenic shock, so blood volume must be restored rapidly with the infusion of fluids and cardiopulmonary resuscitation (CPR) started at the same time, while preferably another team should direct their attention to the airway.

In the absence of expert infrastructure or personnel, cardiac massage may be started right away after checking for the absence of the carotid pulsations. Five rounds (5 s) of cardiac massage may then be followed by an airway check. "Head tilt and chin lift" is the standard procedure for mouth opening and may be performed in all cases by even lay persons with a basic idea about first aid. However, when a cervical spine injury is suspected, as is quite common in case of trauma involving the head and neck region, the "jaw thrust" is the initial procedure of choice. This requires skilled personnel to execute and is not recommended to be undertaken by lay persons involved in the resuscitation of a trauma victim. Mouth-to-mouth ventilation, bag-mask (or Ambu bag or face mask to mouth) ventilation, insertion of an oropharyngeal airway and bagging, using a laryngeal mask or combitube, orotracheal or nasotracheal intubation, and finally a surgical airway or tracheotomy are the usual order in which the airway is established. Any one of these may suffice or a surgical airway may be the first choice in some cases where a known airway obstruction exists or is anticipated.

A full body trauma assessment is a standard part of the ATLS protocol. It assigns a score for injury severity according to the location of injury. The injury severity score (ISS) thus calculated is used as guide for triaging and further management. An ISS of more than 16 is considered extremely grave and requires urgent intervention.

History taking and head and neck examination must be complete and comprehensive. Bone and soft tissue trauma, missing teeth, and impacted objects must be carefully looked for besides attention to the immediate resuscitation of the patient. The first inspection, like the first impression, is the best one and is undertaken as soon as the patient is stable or even concomitantly, especially in cases where the airway must be cleared and circulation established.

Infection control is implied in the management of any kind of trauma. This is important because many a time it is seen that the complications of trauma treatment outstrip the initial management of acute trauma.

Wound management must follow the surgical principles of cleansing, removal of embedded debris and necrotic tissue (debridement), insertion of drain(s) wherever dependent collection or contamination is present or anticipated, antibiotic prophylaxis as and when necessary, administration of tetanus toxoid vaccine where contamination has occurred and in the absence of prior immunization, and careful inspection and documentation of the details of the wound. Clean wounds may be closed primarily provided there is no or minimal tissue loss, unnecessary exposure and other incisions may be avoided wherever possible, and the facial skeleton must be restored as early as possible to avoid scarring and contracture that might eventually compromise essential physiological functions such as eating and speaking. Delayed closure is done when significant collateral damage is present, when other serious injuries take precedence, or when the prognosis is extremely poor. Care of bites and lacerations is carried out with the help of topical medications, wound dressings, and appropriate immunization, for example, administration of anti-rabies vaccine in the case of dog bite or anti-gas gangrene immunoglobulin in the case of severe contamination and/or presence of gas-forming organisms.

Bony disruptions must be managed by plating, which must meet the immediate objective of facial reconstruction as well as the long-term objectives of stability and restoration of normal function. Stability at the fracture site(s) must be ensured by three-point fixation wherever needed and good contact between the fragments. The use of dynamic compression plates (DCP) is popular but not as central to the treatment as in the case of long bone immobilization.

2.3   Medicolegal Aspects

Medicolegal aspects of trauma are extremely important to bear in mind because medical reports and medical certificates often need to be prepared accurately for the purpose of filing insurance claims, compensation, and litigation suits. In addition, when disputes occur, doctors are called as expert witnesses in the court of law, and crucial decisions are made on the basis of such testimony.

1. A *wound* is defined as a breach in the anatomical continuity of a skin surface or mucosal membrane, with or without involvement of the deeper tissue. A wound is produced when the tissue succumbs to external forces of compression, traction, or torsion and is dependent on the mass and velocity of the external agent and the structure of the tissue impacted.
2. An *abrasion* is defined as injury to only the epidermis or outermost layer of the skin caused by a frictional force in either the horizontal or vertical direction, sometimes leaving an imprint of the offending object.
3. A *bruise* is an extravascular accumulation of blood in the subcutaneous layers of the skin and is visible from the outside. A similar entity when not visible externally, for example, when occurring over mucosal surfaces, is called a contusion. A bruise or contusion may be further referred to as petechia, purpura, ecchymosis, or hematoma depending on its size from smallest to largest.
4. A *laceration* is defined as a tear of the skin, mucosa, or viscera due to impact from a blunt force, allowing blood to escape to the exterior of the body or body cavity.
5. A *fracture* is a disruption in the continuity of a bony surface, structure, or organ such as the bone or tooth.
6. An *incised wound* is defined as a clean wound with regular edges caused by a sharp edge applied to the skin in a perpendicular or oblique direction. A slash wound has more length than depth while a stab wound has more depth than length. A stab wound may be further classified as a puncture or penetrating wound. Firearm wounds, blast wounds, and burns and scalds cause a combination of different types of wound due to the characteristics and constituents of the offending material.

Careful assessment of the dentition is very important for the trauma surgeon. While loose, lost, or impacted teeth pose obvious problems for the patient, they also provide vital clues in the event of medicolegal cases and suspected foul play, especially where death has occurred. While the surgeon in this instance does not play an active role in the management of the patient, but an equally important and central role in the criminal investigation process, he or she must not take this role lightly. Reporting on the dentition using the standard representation of the full adult dentition of eight teeth per quadrant numbered from medial to lateral, starting with the right upper and then proceeding to the left upper then followed by the left lower and finally the right lower quadrant, is a crucial part of documentation of the injury. Abnormalities of the teeth such as spacing, number, shape, and size must be carefully documented, preferably with good clinical photographs using standardized methods, such as the use of the ABFO (American Board of Forensic Odontology) scale. The teeth not only furnish information about the age of the patient but also the sex by the presence of Barr bodies in the nucleus of the cells in the soft and hard tissues. The dental cementum incremental rate provides a precise idea of not only the age but also the season or time of year that the victim died. DNA analysis can be performed on the teeth using the polymerase chain reaction (PCR) method and the blood group determined from the salivary fluid obtained from the deceased, even if only traces are found.

The impact of trauma may be manifest as bleeding, shock, airway obstruction, loss of consciousness or loss of function, infection, and permanent disability. Thus, injuries may be known as simple or non-grievous injuries when a wound or bodily damage is caused without serious consequences and grievous injuries when loss of life, limb, or function occurs. Some variations may occur and range from endangering injuries to fatal injuries to include the gamut of simple and grievous injuries.

Medicolegal and ethical issues abound in ENT trauma. One of the principal concerns when dealing with any trauma is whether one is doing the right thing—technically and also morally, legally, and ethically. The implications of this are enormous. Many a time, a doctor carries out a procedure in the best interest of the patient without attention to important issues such as documentation, investigation of the cause, mode or background of the trauma, and, of course, personal safety.

Medicolegal and ethical dilemmas could be encountered when dealing with:

(a) Self-inflicted injury as in suicidal attempts or psychiatric illness, children with foreign bodies
(b) Domestic or family violence
(c) Prisons, shelters, homes, and orphanages
(d) Humanitarian conflicts and war zones
(e) Industrial and occupational trauma
(f) Accidents, natural disasters, and mass casualties
(g) Iatrogenic trauma and medical negligence

Examples of each of the above are:

(a) Epistaxis due to attention-seeking behavior, acid or alkali burns to the face and aerodigestive tract, and foreign bodies
(b) Traumatic perforations; strangulation, throttling, or hanging; and nasal fractures
(c) Hanging, facial and nasal fractures, temporal bone trauma, and foreign bodies in ears (live insects for torture)
(d) Blast injuries, shrapnel and gunshot wounds, and penetrating neck and face injuries
(e) Noise-induced hearing loss (calculate handicap), septal perforation in chemical factories, neck injury due to machinery, airway burns in laboratories, barotraumas in divers and jet pilots, and voice abuse
(f) Head and neck trauma, head injury, and polytrauma
(g) Complications of FESS (functional endoscopic sinus surgery) (anterior ethmoidal artery, lamina papyracea, optic nerve, anterior skull base), mastoid surgery (facial nerve, stapes, LSSC (lateral semicircular canal), jugular bulb, tegmen, sinus plate), throat and airway surgery such as tonsillectomy and adenoidectomy (rough

technique, atlantoaxial dislocation), tracheotomy (pneumothorax, brachiocephalic vein avulsion), thyroid surgery (recurrent laryngeal nerve and parathyroid injury), and intubation (stenosis, web, granuloma, cord paralysis, and dislocation/subluxation)

It is commonly seen that due to the acute exacerbation of an underlying condition following trauma, the patient is highly distressed and seeks instant remedy by operation. This is more likely in cases where foul play has occurred and the aggrieved party has filed a medicolegal case with a view to seeking increased compensation or justice or both.

Surgery in such instances should be deferred for at least 3–4 weeks and preferably 6–8 weeks, in order to allow stabilization of the acute injury and organization of the scar or callus and thus minimize blood loss during surgery. Exceptions are reduction of a nasal bone fracture, suturing of a pinna laceration, or decompression of the facial nerve in case of bony impingement. One must realize that optimal surgical results for the treatment of the primary cause are only possible once the effects of acute injury have worn off. Edema, congestion, granulation tissue, and infection are other reasons why definitive surgery may have to be postponed. This would also allow better evaluation of the social, financial, and legal aspects of the traumatic event with regard to the primary lesion. Counseling and supportive care are imperative during this period. Though it might be difficult to sustain a patient's motivation for definitive surgical treatment till an optimal point in time, it should be impressed upon the patient and the family that this is being done only in their best interests and for no other reason.

Legal and ethical considerations should take into account that disclosure is sometimes not only permissible but also compulsory. The Data Protection Act, Mental Capacity Act, codes of professional conduct, matters pertaining to the interest of public health, and the presence of advance directives if any must be borne in mind. A quick screen for telltale criminal behavior is important and should be an instinctive part of the initial evaluation of a trauma patient, such as may happen when a dangerous or lethal weapon is probably being concealed. Many a time, a trauma patient may refuse emergency care by forgetting or being ignorant of the serious and irreversible consequences of doing the same. The presence of intoxication, head injury, hypoxia, mental illness, old age, and dementia may be found to interfere with the ability of the patient to make a decision, but it must not be mistaken for diminished mental capacity. Enough time and opportunity must be given to the patient till he or she is in a state of mind to make a rational decision regarding his or her treatment. Paperwork and relevant documentation are extremely important in order to safeguard the medicolegal aspects of trauma management. Advance directives (ADs) or living wills must be interpreted in the appropriate context and not necessarily applied to all situations in order to ensure the well-being of the patient.

It is imperative to distinguish between ethics and the law and important to remember that following the law does not necessarily result in ethical behavior, and conversely, ethical behavior may not always be protected by the law. However, it is often difficult to distinguish between the two as far as management of trauma is concerned. The outcomes of legal and ethical considerations, though similar, may differ greatly if analyzed in the theoretical context. Thus, the situation varies greatly from case to case, and both medical professionals and their patients are served best by utmost care in the documentation of the proceedings and in communication with the patient's family and also law enforcement officers, taking cognizance of the fact that all the parties involved are competent enough to make and execute decisions.

The four tenets of ethical behavior must be followed at all times, and these include beneficence, justice, non-maleficence, and autonomy. All this involves rapid decision making and procedural skills, the capacity for which usually comes from experience but also gleaned in considerable measure by correct and sustained training. The provision of care must be accompanied by correct and relevant documentation in the form of medical records and followed up with periodic audit and review. Clinical dilemmas and the research aspects of trauma often spill over from the emergency center into the intensive care unit and operation theater. As the patient is often in alien and unfamiliar surroundings, far removed from his or her usual medical or insurance provider, there are high levels of frustration, stress, and anxiety. The emergency care provider is often not aware of pre-existing conditions and not in a condition to obtain an adequate medical history, and so the chances of errors and subsequent complications are very high indeed. It is also immensely difficult to gain the patient's confidence and establish a rapport with the patient. Expensive and life-saving equipment is very often employed to provide care to trauma patients without prejudice, and consideration of reimbursement or outcomes, and thus the management of trauma, is a labor-intensive and perhaps not economically viable option in many trauma centers. Consent is often tacit and implied and not always expressed, complicating decision making and leading to legal hassles later.

Multiple providers increase the risk of missing other injuries, especially those which fall outside the purview of a particular specialty. It is worthwhile remembering that access to emergency care services is a basic human right; thus, any emergency department (ED) worth its name must be well equipped if legal sanctions are to be avoided. Special cases include sexual assault, drug-related injuries, elder or child abuse, and interpersonal family violence. Meticulous documentation is imperative, and recalling things and events from memory, especially following a tense situation, is not even a close substitute for a careful and detailed clinical record done in real time.

A range of conditions from minor to life-threatening may exist, and the patient may not disclose many personal details, leading health practitioners to practice excessive use of personal protection, which understandably causes an unpleasant experience for the patient. The chances of the patient having committed an offense or concealing a weapon pose considerable risk to staff, but an investigation of the same may be resisted on the grounds of invasion of privacy. Continuation of care may be futile in many cases but disputed or argued in either direction by different members of the patient's family. Thus it is prudent to follow the principle of acting in the patient's best interest, and sometimes it may be necessary to take recourse to other options such as proxy consent and substituted judgment. The risk of liability

Table 2.1 Trauma protocols at a glance (category at bottom in bold italics)

Time	Triage	Black	Primary survey	Airway	Beneficence
Place	Airway	Red	Resuscitation	Breathing	Justice
Nature	Imaging	Amber	Secondary survey	Circulation	Non-maleficence
Costs	Trauma Team	Yellow	Definitive care	Disability	Autonomy
Rehabilitation		Green		Exposure	
		Blue			
General considerations	*Polytrauma*	*Triage color coding*	*ATLS protocol*	*Components of primary survey*	*Ethics and law*

includes vicarious liability, and the standard of care is as per the reasonable practitioner approach.

Different countries across the world have designated sections in their penal code signifying the type of injury and the penalty or punishment thereof, and a detailed discussion of the same is beyond the scope of this book.

The different aspects of trauma protocols are summarized in Table 2.1.

2.4   Practical Applications

Very often in the management of trauma, there may arise the need to use blood and blood products such as packed red cells, platelets, fresh frozen plasma, and cryoprecipitate, depending on what deficiency in the circulation it requires to be fulfilled. Whole fresh blood, stored blood, and packed red cells with additives are used to make up severe blood loss in hemorrhagic conditions. The risk of infection and contamination is high with fresh whole blood; thus, it is always better to use blood that has been safely tested and stored under optimum conditions. Voluntary blood donation should be encouraged. It may not be essential to use whole blood in all cases, and blood components be just as useful, for example, fresh frozen plasma (FFP) can be used when trauma is complicated by systemic problems such as disseminated intravascular coagulation (DIC) or coagulopathies. FFP contains factors 8 and 12, von Willebrand's factor, fibronectin, and fibrinogen. Similarly, cryoprecipitate may be used when pre-existing conditions such as hypofibrinogenemia or afibrinogenemia exist.

2.4.1   Complications of Transfusion

Complications of transfusion of blood or blood products include chills, pulmonary edema, volume overload, acute kidney injury, HLA alloimmunization or graft versus host disease (GVHD), viral transmission, bacterial infection, and allergic reactions. According to recent guidelines, blood products need to be given if the hemoglobin (Hb) is less than 8 g percent, and not 10 g percent as was earlier the norm. Also, any elective procedure in the management of trauma may be done with the administration of oral iron, a semi-elective one with iron injections, an emergency with packed red cells, or blood component, and whole blood may be reserved for only a dire emergency.

As far as possible, blood or blood products should be given only after grouping and crossmatching, and the earlier practice of using "O" blood as a "universal donor," even though acceptable in a dire emergency, is no longer recommended under the current ATLS protocols.

The international normalized ratio (INR) should be optimized to 1.5 before any neurosurgical procedure such as a craniotomy or burr hole, but an INR of up to 2.0 is acceptable before an invasive surgical procedure. As a rule of thumb, any mucosal bleed or a platelet count below 25,000 should be managed with a platelet transfusion.

Methods of minimizing or completely avoiding a blood transfusion include predonation, hypotensive epidural analgesia, normovolemic hemodilution, autologous capture and transfusion, surgical treatment or direct arrest of bleeding, prevention of bleeding (by anticipation and preparation), local infiltration of anesthetic agents and vasoconstrictors, observance of meticulous technique, and use of local hemostatic agents (thrombotic agents, platelet gels, fibrin sealants, tranexamic acid, botropase, and epsilon aminocaproic acid—EACA).

While it is fairly easy to assess the amount of obvious or visible blood loss, the trauma physician or surgeon must also bear in mind invisible blood loss, or that which might be taking place inside a body compartment and is therefore not obvious. This is particularly important in the case of polytrauma and is likely to happen in the case of concomitant head, pelvic, thoracic, or abdominal injury. A thorough physical examination of the whole patient is therefore of utmost importance, regardless of which specialty is primarily called upon to manage the trauma patient.

Though the body has four times the reserve capacity for blood loss, it is incumbent upon any practitioner of trauma, and at any level, to be able to swiftly gauge the gravity of the situation. The Glasgow Coma Scale (GCS) should be at the fingertips of any medical professional while assessing the extent of traumatic brain injury (TBI) as this would be the crucial decision maker as to whether the patient will live or die. A GCS of less than 8/15 mandates an airway support with the help of endotracheal intubation. Each successive physician or surgeon, while taking a handoff or answering a consultation, must confirm the GCS score and make or alter a decision based on current and updated assessments.

In disasters and mass casualties, surgeons from various disciplines may be called upon to deal with victims of trauma. It is usually seen that in such instances, surgeons of different specialties limit themselves to the region of their expertise, but many a time there may be an overlap. For example, otolaryngologists are intimately familiar with facial injuries, but so are plastic and reconstructive surgeons. Though first aid and primary management can be carried out by either one, the higher specialty should naturally take over when a difficulty or complication is encountered, if such services are available in the immediate or nearby location. Failure to ensure this may result in medicolegal hassles and delay in the treatment of the patient.

Of late, more and more emphasis is being placed on digitization of patient-related information and the use of electronic medical records (EMR) and electronic health records (EHR). It is crucial to maintain accurate details of a trauma event in such records not only for the proper treatment to be carried out at each level, and often at the different places that the patient might receive treatment, but also for medicolegal purposes, such as when giving evidence in a court of law. Countries adopting a green policy and switching to a completely paperless system are now allowing electronic information of patients to be provided in a court of law. However, a good number of these also maintain parallel paper records where minute and essential details are documented. This is especially relevant in case of patients suffering from chronic disease, psychiatric illness, and sexually transmitted diseases. In the event of a trauma, such details may be missing and may interfere with the comprehensive management of the patient.

2.4.2 Documentation

Documentation is crucial to the optimal management of trauma. As anatomical structure is distorted by trauma, clinical photographs taken in correct scientific orientation help not only to understand the mechanism by which the trauma has occurred but also how to plan treatment. Comparison with previous photographs of the patient when healthy helps to predict the extent and outcome of surgical correction and sets realistic expectations. This is extremely important in order to avoid patient dissatisfaction and the inclination to seek legal remedy if the treatment does not produce the outcome desired. Documentation is thus extremely important even in the case of such exigencies and not just in planned, cold, and elective cases.

Clinical photographs are an important source of information as documentation is required not only for medical and academic purposes but also for the purpose of insurance, legal matters, and future follow-up. The services of a professional photographer are desirable and indeed mandatory for many settings, though photographic documentation may also be done on personal devices such as mobile phones, digital cameras, and laptop computers by individual practitioners.

Documentation in trauma may suffer from the recording of minute but important details because of the urgency of the situation and lack of time. Nevertheless, it is crucial to maintain medical records for not only the immediate management of the patient but also to fulfill medicolegal and insurance purposes as well as future follow-up. Modern devices such as electronic medical records, with or without the help of speech recognition software and implements in the form of Dictaphone, go a long way in maintaining detailed documentation. Reports of investigations and treatment records, especially of surgeries planned and done, are the areas most benefitted by the use of efficient hospital information management systems (HIMS) with the above facilities.

2.4.3 Communication

Communication with the patient, family, as well as friends and bystanders who might have brought a trauma victim to a healthcare facility is also central to a smooth treatment and rehabilitation process and avoidance of insurance and medicolegal hassles. This is indeed a tall order given the emergent nature of managing trauma and the need to innovate and improvise according to the situation at hand. Combined with proper documentation, clear communication helps to expedite and optimize the management of a trauma victim.

2.4.4 Antibiotic Policy

Antibiotic policy is a major concern in trauma practice. Surgeons by and large are wary of antibiotics and antimicrobial resistance, on the one hand, and compelled to use multiple antibiotics in the face of complicated trauma. Unlike elective surgery, it is almost impossible to prevent contamination and risk of infection when dealing with trauma, except in certain cases of iatrogenic trauma.

Antimicrobial drugs may be used by surgeons for the prevention of wound infection and also for its treatment. These two kinds of use vary greatly in nature and magnitude. The instances in which trauma surgeons need to be cognizant of antibiotic use, especially in the case of wound infection prophylaxis, lie in several parameters. The most important one is to determine the benefits of prophylactic antibiotic use against its inherent risks. Obviously, this would depend on the general health and physical condition of the patient, as determined by the trauma surgeon and graded according to the ASA (American Society of Anesthesiologists) criteria. Another crucial factor in determining risk is the status of the wound, in other words, whether it is clean, contaminated, clean-contaminated, or dirty, as is popularly practiced.

The extent or magnitude of the operative procedure, in other words the amount and depth of tissue involved, plays a major role in selecting an antibiotic for prophylaxis or whether or not prophylaxis is required at all. The further choice of the antibiotic depends on whether the tissue concerned is compatible for the antibiotic, for example, quinolones such as ciprofloxacin penetrate cartilage well, whereas clindamycin is suitable for the salivary glands. The time of scheduling of the surgery and also its duration are further determinants of the use of a prophylactic antibiotic. It is best administered as close as possible to the time of taking the first incision, and a procedure of long duration may require more than one dose of prophylaxis.

Antimicrobial resistance (*AMR*) arises due to indiscriminate use by physicians, practitioners of veterinary medicine, and use in various types of industry. In many developing countries, public sector hospitals dispense antibiotics depending upon the availability of current stock and government policies pertaining to that region, which may or may not be along recommended and expected guidelines. Doctors are not uniform in their use of antibiotics, in many instances owing to ignorance and absence of a culture of evidence based practice. Dogma and profiteering by individual doctors and pharmacists also play no mean role in the emergence of antimicrobial resistance. Patients' demands, a lack of confidence in the results of laboratory investigations, traditional beliefs, half-baked knowledge and lack of trust in doctors, easy availability of over-the-counter (OTC) medications, aggressive marketing by the pharmaceutical industry, the growing popularity of online purchase (e.g., azithromycin), and consultation are the myriad of ways that resistance to antibiotics is growing by the day and posing a threat to human life. More than anything, it is in the treatment of trauma that many of these considerations must be borne in mind because the patient is often forced to seek treatment in a place that is unfamiliar, and much of these factors might be overlooked. Wound infection then becomes a much more challenging problem to deal with than the mere management of the acute trauma itself. A useful way to deal with this is to opt for a topical preparation whenever applicable.

2.5   Future Directions

2.5.1   Trauma as a Subspecialist Discipline

Trauma as a subspecialist discipline started in 2007 and was based on the management of mass casualties and disasters, using ethical and scientific principles of triage, in other words providing comfort care for those who were deemed unsalvageable. It thus includes both operative and nonoperative care and graduated levels of care such as intensive care unit (ICU) and high dependency unit (HDU). Trainees of various levels of skill and experience and the influx or migration of medical professionals from different ethnicities, cultures, and philosophies mean that chaos and confusion often rule in many trauma services and trauma centers. The concept of damage control surgery has resulted in staggered and multiple operative procedures, often at the hands of different providers, complicating care and making the provision of trauma services extremely exasperating for most patients. While the decision to withhold or withdraw life support is a medical one, political and cultural factors may play a major role and confound the situation greatly.

2.5.2   Recovery from Trauma

Recovery from trauma involves tissue regeneration and restoration of normal function. This is always desirable but at the same time unpredictable in certain situations and also dependent on various factors surrounding the trauma episode. At times, tissue regeneration can go haywire and result in unsightly scarring and loss of function, as seen in facial deformity and airway stenosis. Experimental studies are now focused on the recognition of agents that are crucial to tissue repair and renewal and the use of antagonistic agents that could help to keep florid and uncontrollable repair processes under check. One of these is the anti-vascular endothelial growth factor or anti-VEGF. While the use of this is tested and tried in malignancies like renal cell and colon carcinoma, research is on for use of the same in trauma and various other diseases. Platelet-rich plasma, mesenchymal stem cells, and hepatocyte growth factor show promising results as well in both "in vitro" and "in vivo" models [3–6].

2.5.3 Research in Trauma Care

Research in trauma care is thus extremely daunting and often controlled tightly by the laws of the state. Most research in trauma is in the area of experimental basic research on the one hand and minimally invasive observational research on the other because the authority to waive consent or use delayed consent is not available to trauma service providers. This naturally deters useful and practical research, such as that into newer modalities of treatment like devices, procedures, and even drugs. Institutional mandate for ethical review makes any research beyond retrospective case series and audits cumbersome, and taking the research protocol through all the necessary steps is daunting for most trauma practitioners. The high prevalence of the human immunodeficiency virus (HIV) and the HIV opt-out testing facility has improved the safety profile for doctors dealing with trauma and research in this area.

Conclusion

Even though trauma is unpredictable, sudden, and very often life-threatening, specific principles and guidelines must always be borne in mind. These must be applied as per the demands of a particular situation, all the time keeping in mind the medicolegal problems which may prove daunting in many cases.

References

1. Thrall JH. Radiation exposure in CT scanning and risk: where are we? Radiology. 2012;264:325–8
2. Masaryk T, Kolonick R, Painter T, Weinreb DB. The economics and clinical benefits of portable head/neck CT imaging in the intensive care unit. Radiol Manage. 2008;30(2):50–4
3. Sclafani AP, Azzi J. Platelet preparations for use in facial rejuvenation and wound healing: a critical review of current literature. Aesthet Plast Surg. 2015;39:495–505
4. Woo SH, Jeong HS, Kim JP, Koh EH, Lee SU, Jin SM, et al. Favorable vocal fold wound healing induced by platelet-rich plasma injection. Clin Exp Otorhinolaryngol. 2014;7:47–52
5. Cho HH, Jang S, Lee SC, Jeong HS, Park JS, Han JY, et al. Effect of neural-induced mesenchymal stem cells and platelet rich plasma on facial nerve regeneration in an acute nerve injury model. Laryngoscope. 2010;120:907–13
6. Xu CC, Chan RW, Weinberger DG, Efune G, Pawlowski KS. Controlled release of hepatocyte growth factor from a bovine acellular scaffold for vocal fold reconstruction. J Biomed Mater Res A. 2010;93(4):1335–47

Injury and Wound Healing

> **Learning Objectives**
> - To understand the cellular basis of tissue injury and wound healing
> - To consider the mechanism of injury when dealing with particular cases of trauma
> - To remember important principles that determine outcomes in trauma

3.1 Wound Healing

3.1.1 Zones of Perfusion

Normal healing is dependent on sufficient blood supply to the skin and subcutaneous tissues according to the zones of perfusion. These zones are:

1. Zone I—the systemic circulation supported by the cardiopulmonary system
2. Zone II—the capillary circulation at the level of the tissue and overlying skin
3. Zone III—the interstitial spaces
4. Zone IV—the cells and cell membranes

The vitality of the above levels of perfusion may be assessed on the basis of the patient's history, personal history pertaining to habits and vices such as smoking and alcohol abuse, medical conditions such as hypertension and diabetes mellitus, physical examination, and general condition, all of which would help to determine not only the prognosis and natural healing process but also the relative risks of surgical intervention and anesthesia.

Once trauma has occurred and a wound has formed, the natural tendency of the body is to aid in its healing. Several factors come into play at this stage—the site and extent of the wound, its depth and the involvement of the underlying or nearby structures, the loss of normal tissue if any, and of course, the mechanism of

© Springer Nature Singapore Pte Ltd. 2018

J. Das, *Trauma in Otolaryngology*, https://doi.org/10.1007/978-981-10-6361-9_3

injury—whether the wound is caused by a clean incision or an avulsion crush injury. Other important factors are whether contamination by impacted foreign bodies or debris is present or bacterial infection due to microorganisms has occurred. The general condition of the patient and the state of the immune system are important factors for prognosis. For example, a concomitant viral infection causing general debility and medical comorbidities such as anemia, diabetes mellitus or cardiovascular disease, or an underlying malignancy or HIV infection, cancer chemotherapy or radiotherapy, or the chronic use of oral corticosteroids for any reason, could all greatly influence the capacity of the body to help in the spontaneous resolution of a wound caused by trauma. Habits such as smoking or alcohol abuse could cause further problems such as vascular compromise due to microangiopathy or major vessel disease causing arterial or venous insufficiency and poor nutritional status causing malnutrition and deficiency of vitamins, minerals, and micronutrients. The position of a dependent part and the use of trusses, collars, or bulky bandages could further worsen venous congestion, vascular insufficiency, and the tendency to develop a pressure or decubitus ulcer.

3.1.2   Healing and Closure of Wounds

This may be by primary, secondary, or tertiary intention. Healing by primary intention occurs when the edges of the wound are opposed precisely. It leaves a minimal scar and is thus called normal healing. Healing by secondary intention occurs when the wound edges cannot be opposed, and therefore the wound is left open. Inflammatory reactions and hyperemia or increased vascular flow causes proliferation of granulation tissue which later undergoes epithelization and contracts, resulting in a visible or obvious scar. A combination of the above two may be understood as healing by tertiary intention. In this the wound edges may not be opposed, and the site may require cleaning, dressing, and debridement until granulation tissue starts to appear and the wound starts to contract. At this point, the edges could be brought closer together and sutured so as to hasten the healing process and optimize the resulting scar. Thus this is also known as delayed primary intention.

Wound healing can be understood better with the knowledge of skin tissue anatomy and physiology and adequate blood flow through the tissue at all times. The vascular components are made up of red blood cells, neutrophils, platelets, macrophages, and reticulocytes. The lining of the blood vessels also contributes by way of endothelial cells and vascular smooth muscle. The tissue components are the dermis with fibroblasts and myofibroblasts; the adnexal organs such as dermal papilla cells surrounding the hair follicles and the outer root sheath cells; the epidermal elements composed of melanocytes, keratinocytes, and Langerhans cells; the subcutaneous adipose tissue and fat cells; and last but not the least, the neuroendocrine regulation of blood circulation through neurons and hormones.

During the healing process, two distinct stages can be observed. The first one is the stage of inflammation where platelet-derived growth factor (PDGF), epidermal growth factor (EGF), and transforming growth factor (TGF)-beta are expressed.

These then attract keratinocytes which migrate to the site of injury and proliferate, allowing regeneration of a new epithelium, and this stage is known as the stage of proliferation. Both these processes take place in the early phase of trauma, namely, 2–3 days, and result in granulation tissue formation, with fibroblasts entering the site and releasing hyaluronic acid and fibronectin, which constitute the immature form of granulation tissue. This is the scaffold which serves as the foundation for the migration and adherence of more fibroblasts, and this is responsible for the formation of the dermal matrix that helps in the production of collagen types 1 and 3. Angiogenesis also occurs at the same time with the help of aFGF (FGF-1) and bFGF (FGF-2)—the acid and base varieties of the angiogenic fibroblast growth factor.

As more days elapse, the wound starts to contract, with the continued expression of TGF-beta which leads to fibroblasts producing alpha smooth muscle actin. This is also evident histologically by the appearance of alpha smooth muscle actin as seen with its increased propensity to take up stain. In experimental animals such as mice, this has been observed to occur between 15 and 30 days after injury. The stage of remodeling then follows, and this eventually restores the elasticity of the skin up to 80% of the normal. This is mainly due to the continuous replacement of type 3 collagen by type 1 collagen until the normal ratio of 1:4 (type 3 to 1) has been achieved. So the natural healing process is capable of restoring almost full structure and function to the injured site.

The first step in trauma management is obviously immediate treatment of the wound. Again, factors such as nature and extent of injury are crucial in order to decide how to proceed with wound management. The wound may have to be cleansed and debrided to allow a thorough exploration and to determine what needs to be done further. At this stage, even a working diagnosis must be made that would define the line of treatment to be followed, for example, "a single incised wound over the auricle with exposure of cartilage" or "an external deformity of the nose with fracture of the nasal bones and septal hematoma." Damaged tissues and structures must then be repaired or corrected, and the timing for doing so must be planned carefully. Relevant investigations may have to be undertaken, such as basic blood and laboratory tests, and plain X-rays at the minimum. Loss of tissue should be restored wherever possible to maintain cosmetic and esthetic appearance, and physiological function, but not at the expense of compromised viability and risk of infection and necrosis. Similarly, the overlying skin should be assessed for viability and the possibility of closure without unnecessary tension or stretching of the skin. Undermining of the edges of the wound may be done to reduce tension and allow adequate closure for suturing. If parts of the skin cover are missing, consideration should be given to skin grafts and free or pedicled flaps. Needless to say, such decisions must be accompanied by delicate handling of tissue and good surgical technique based on sound medical evidence. Evidence-based practice in emergency practice such as trauma may not always be possible as surgeons continuously improvise according to the situation, but here evidence-based surgery mainly refers to the many controversies regarding management of individual injuries which have been discussed throughout this text in the relevant chapters and is aimed not at the emergent treatment of trauma but at improving outcomes of trauma management.

Nevertheless, it is important to remember that the natural healing process can be greatly enhanced by proper attention to wound care and preparation for the outcome of a minimal scar and external deformity. If the skin is allowed to heal by primary intention, sound techniques of skin closure need to be meticulously followed. First of all, closure should always be done along the natural relaxed skin tension lines (RSTL), but this may not always be possible and other techniques have to be followed. These include close coaptation and good alignment of the wound edges. If much tissue has been lost and it is difficult to bring the margins together, undermining of the edges may be done so that closure can be carried out without undue tension after suturing. Vertical mattress sutures with nonabsorbable suture materials and using buried subcutaneous sutures with absorbable materials also help.

Once the wound has been cleaned and closed, the next step is to wait for healing to occur. Antibiotics and anti-inflammatory medication, antacids, vitamins, and so on, along with rest, proper diet, exercise, and physiotherapy wherever required, must be instituted according to the need of the patient and the general condition and/ or the presence of other injuries or medical comorbidities. One must be vigilant for the signs of impending infection and wound breakdown. Pain may be masked by medication, so the presence of pain and tenderness is an early sign of infection. Fever is usually absent due to the administration of antibiotics and analgesics/anti-pyretic drugs. There may be increased redness of the wound edges and involvement of the surrounding skin by edema and induration—an early sign of cellulitis. Subcutaneous emphysema due to gas gangrene should be ruled out clinically, as also the presence of blisters over the skin signifying the appearance of vacuoles and wound necrosis.

Discoloration of the skin, areas of blackening suggesting necrosis or gangrene, pallor and absence of pulsations, and the appearance of "dishwater pus"—a gray-colored discharge from the wound—are late manifestations of infection and generally spell doom for the survival of the tissue. The release of toxins and inflammatory mediators from such a necrotic wound leads to their spillover into the circulation and subsequent septicemia, coagulopathy, hypovolemic and endotoxic shock, renal shutdown, and ultimately multiorgan failure.

For good and timely healing to occur, the blood circulation in the tissue or organ must be maintained at a careful balance. Trauma can lead to disturbances in both the arterial supply and venous drainage. While deficiencies in the arterial supply may be seen as pallor of the skin over the affected part or attenuation of the skin by shriveling or thinning, stasis or venous congestion due to impaired drainage would manifest as a dark discoloration of the skin with attendant turgidity or bulkiness. The same changes tend to affect a skin flap or free tissue transfer done for coverage and reconstruction of the wound.

The viability of the arterial circulation is crucial for good wound healing and survival of local or free flaps and is therefore more important than the venous stasis, if any. Venous stasis may however add to the problem of deficient arterial circulation and must be avoided at all costs. Ischemia is usually not tolerated for more than 12 h, unless favorable conditions exist such as induced hypothermia or the use of crystalloid solutions to maintain circulatory volume with relative hemodilution.

Increased tendency for coagulation can occur as a result of injury to the tissue and its blood vessels and also the presence of systemic changes such as sepsis or DIC (disseminated intravascular coagulation), and any of these may exacerbate the poor blood supply to the tissue in addition to the blood loss suffered by the traumatic event.

The use of heparinized blood, colloids such as dextran, and medications such as aspirin helps to increase vascular supply and maintain viability of tissue. Heparin inhibits factors 5 and 8 and thus has an antithrombotic effect. It may be used as heparinized lidocaine or saline, the former more useful when repairing wounds under local anesthesia. Dextran acts as an anticoagulant by inhibiting and degrading fibrin while also being a tissue and plasma expander. Aspirin acts by inhibition of the cyclooxygenase pathway and decreases thromboxane while increasing prostacy-clins, thus facilitating increased blood flow.

A poorly healed skin scar may be corrected by excising and resuturing it or by excising it and inserting a skin expander if the defect is too large and the skin edges cannot be aligned together. In the latter case, some time must elapse before the final suturing can be done. Other tried and tested methods are doing a Z-plasty, W-plasty, or geometric broken line closure (GBLC). These are known as irregularization techniques. Resurfacing can also be done using dermabrasion. These are especially important in the face and neck regions in order to avoid an ugly and visible scar.

While definitive surgical scar revision is being contemplated, temporary methods such as wigs and hairpieces, spectacles, makeup styles, and prosthetic appliances may be used to tide over the patient's functional and social handicap [1]. Such measures can be used soon after the primary injury and repair up to 6–12 months later until the scar has matured and is ready for revision. It also affords the patient valuable time to decide on future course of action and final appearance depending on the functional deficit perceived.

Apart from a poorly healed scar, the other common problem is dealing with hypertrophic and keloidal scars. A hypertrophic scar, as the name suggests, is an exuberantly healed scar with overexpression of fibrotic tissue but that which tends to remain static and confined to the edges of the wound. A keloid scar on the other hand is a scar gone haywire; in other words, it is capable of extending much beyond the original wound and involves considerable amounts of skin in the nearby vicinity. The word keloid is derived from the Greek word "chele" meaning claw or hoof, thus invoking the claw-like and sideways movement of a crab. Though no exact cause is known for either type of abnormal scar, infection plays a major role in the former type, while genetic variations are important in the latter type, as for example, persons of African or Negro origin are predisposed to it compared to Caucasians and Mongoloids.

Steroid injections into the edges of the wound may be tried in people or situations where a hypertrophic or keloid scar is anticipated. For the treatment of established exuberant scars, pressure dressings with customized molds or tightly elasticized coverings or clothes may be tried. Alternatively, aluminum or silicone sheeting may be used along with intralesional injection of the steroid triamcinolone or the application of the antimetabolite colchicine. Radiotherapy using external beam or brachytherapy techniques postoperatively has also been tried, especially for the treatment of keloids. A complete excision of the keloid and secondary suturing of the defect can also be done. A combination of the above techniques, for example, using excision and steroid injection or radiation after the procedure, may have to be done in some cases. Home remedies such as massaging coconut or palm oil, or even vitamin E, are tried by many with or without their doctor's advice, though the efficacy of such treatments has not been scientifically proven. Some scars appear uncommonly red and angry and laser has been tried to reduce such discoloration, but it is likely that this is a part of the natural healing process and does not require any treatment at all.

When revising a scar, debulking is a useful method especially where the scar is hypertrophic or keloidal, leading to a volume excess. Aggressive treatment of such scars may result in recurrence, so the minimal intervention provided by debulking is a sound option [2].

Various other methods of scar revision have been studied, and lasers such as the CO_2 laser are especially useful for minimizing future scarring, but similar results may be obtained with dermabrasion using sterilized drywall sandpaper [3].

Though radiotherapy has been used as a method for revising and improving the appearance of scar tissue, even doses of 15–20 gray over five to six sessions are seen to result in side effects such as erythema and hyperpigmentation if used in the acute postoperative period, and this method greatly increases the risk of radiation-induced malignancy [4].

Large areas of full thickness tissue loss may be restored to almost normal appearance and function with the use of flaps, both local or regional, and distant or free flaps. The use of flaps was first studied in cancer surgery and has evolved over the years to include reconstruction of defects and wounds due to trauma. Flaps must be based on scientific principles such as the vascular pattern of the feeding arteries, layers of tissue and structures required to fill the defect, and methods to ensure survival and function of the flap.

The most crucial of all the above principles is the arterial supply of the flap used for reconstruction. Musculocutaneous arteries are the main mechanism of blood supply to the skin in human beings, and septocutaneous (fasciocutaneous or direct cutaneous) are present in other animals such as cattle, which have principally extensive subcutaneous muscle such as the panniculus carnosus. In human beings, only vestiges of such muscle exist in the form of the platysma in the neck and the dartos in the scrotum.

3.1.3 Flaps

Flaps may be broadly classified into the following:

1. *Random cutaneous flap*—in this the vascular supply is from the subdermal plexus. This is popularly used for reconstruction with local flaps. The plane of dissection is through the subcutaneous fat. The different techniques of using this type of flap

are advancement, rotation, a combination of rotation and advancement, transposition, and the use of tubed flaps. The viability and survival are dependent on the perfusion pressure and not on the length to width ratio. Thus it is imperative to maintain a good systemic circulation when using this kind of flap.

2. *Arterial cutaneous flap*—this is supplied by a defined septocutaneous artery traversing underneath the long axis of the flap. The plane of dissection incorporates the septocutaneous vessel along with the subcutaneous fat. This type of flap is more durable as compared to random flaps as far as survival of the flap is concerned and may be a suitable option in many instances of extensive head and neck trauma. Some examples of this type of flap are the deltopectoral flap which is based on perforators of the internal mammary artery and the paramedian forehead flap which is based on the supratrochlear arteries. Fasciocutaneous flaps such as the parascapular and radial forearm flap may also be used.

3. *Myocutaneous flap*—this has a better outcome in terms of survival of the flap. It is based on the distal segmental vessels and leaves the local vasculature intact but includes muscle also into the flap harvest, lending it more strength and elasticity. Myocutaneous flaps may be known according to the name of the donor muscle used. Examples of such flaps are the pectoralis major myocutaneous (PMMC) flap based on the pectoral branch of the thoracoacromial artery and which forms the workhorse of head and neck cancer surgery and the latissimus dorsi myocutaneous flap that is based on the thoracodorsal artery. This flap design is ideal for wounds that are contaminated or infected.

4. *Free microvascular flap*—this may be a fasciocutaneous, musculocutaneous, myofascial, osseous, or osteocutaneous flap or a combination of any or all of these. It can be tailored to the need of the patient and the size of the wound.

The use of muscle in the flap provides bulk and the bone provides strength, while the skin and mucosa provide sensation. The judicious use of all these elements ensures good structure and function in the repair undertaken. Complex flaps have been traditionally used for the restoration of large defects such as oromandibular and pharyngoesophageal reconstruction in the skull base and pharynx following extirpative surgery for malignancies. They may be safely used in trauma patients who have been irradiated as well for pre-existing malignancy, especially with modern tissue-sparing techniques such as intensity-modulated radiotherapy (IMRT) or image-guided radiotherapy (IGRT).

More popular among the complex flaps are the radial forearm fasciocutaneous flap which is a tubed flap and provides bulk and adynamic swallowing in patients who have lost large areas of the food pipe due to open trauma or burns, and the radial forearm osteocutaneous free flap (OCRFFF). This latter flap is capable of providing 10–15 cm of full thickness tissue and is ideal for reconstruction of the oral cavity and mandible. It is less bulky and more elastic and provides not only a bone template for the endosseous implantation of artificial teeth but is also capable of sensation. It has a long pedicle and is supplied with a sturdy feeding artery. It is possible to harvest this flap at the same sitting and point in time as the primary surgery and results in minimal morbidity at the donor site.

Among the well-known free flaps is the fibula free flap, which is ideal for mandible reconstruction as it can provide a length of bone up to 25 cm, the longest that is possible from a free flap. Other free flaps are the iliac crest flap and the scapular/parascapular flap, but these are associated with variable degrees of donor site morbidity in terms of appearance and function. The rectus abdominis and latissimus dorsi flaps are muscular flaps and are especially useful in pharyngeal repair because they may help to restore swallowing to some extent.

Important physiological considerations in freshly harvested flaps are:

1. *Poor blood supply and the critical closing pressure*—It is possible for a flap to withstand up to 13 h of complete lack of blood supply on an average and still be able to survive. There may be poor blood flow due to the formation of a thrombus at the site of repair, and venous and lymphatic drainage may also be affected, altering physiological dynamics such as Starling's forces, thus further compromising the ischemia.

2. *Microcirculatory changes*—the blood flow may be impaired for prolonged periods of time, leading to lack of nutrition in the flap. Furthermore, hemodynamic disturbances such as sludging and stacking of red blood corpuscles, adhesion of leukocytes, and activation of platelets at the site of the anastomotic repair can also take place. Tearing, stretching, laceration, or crushing of the flap can occur. At the microvascular level, swelling of the endothelial cells and microembolic phenomena can take place.

3. *Neovascularization*—a layer of fibrin forms at the site of repair in the first few days following flap harvest. Formation of new blood vessels, or neovascularization, starts soon afterwards. The establishment of new blood vessels, or revascularization, allows the pedicle of the flap to be divided even as early as 7 days. New capillaries are known to grow from a blood vessel at the rate of 0.2 mm per day on an average. Growth factors that stimulate the growth of new capillaries can help them expand in length up to 2–5 mm. However, pericytes tend to suppress endothelial growth if they come into direct contact with the intima, and are important in the regulation and maturation of new blood vessels. In addition, various substances that affect new blood vessel formation are released by macrophages, lymphocytes, mast cells, and platelets. Autologous or allograft tissues which help to provide growth factors for new vessel formation are the corpus luteum, retina, salivary glands, lymphatic tissues, benign and malignant tumors, and the brain tissue of cows.

4. *Nerve section*—the severance of sensory and symphathetic nerves can greatly affect blood flow in the flap. For example, denervation of the adrenergic supply causes a hyperadrenergic state due to the accumulation of spasm-inducing chemicals at the site of repair, and leads to reduced survival of the flap. If sympathectomy has also been done as part of the procedure or due to the traumatic injury, the resultant vasoconstriction leads to further reduction of the overall blood flow. Only upon depletion of the stored transmitter over the next 24–48 h does the blood flow increase due to reduction in the concentration of norepinephrine.

5. *Products of inflammation*—these are histamine, serotonin, kinins, and prosta-glandins that are released into the circulation once the flap has been elevated. These substances cause increased permeability of the blood vessels at the level of the microcirculation. Proteins and cells accumulate locally in the extracellular compartment and are capable of impairing vascular supply to the flap.

6. *Reperfusion injury*—this is also an important factor to consider. The feeding vessel in the harvested flap (zone 1) may undergo irreversible spasm and cause a no-reflow phenomenon, thereby leading to flap necrosis, while reperfusion injury occurs mainly in zones 2 and 3 due to release and accumulation of free radicals and the mediators of inflammation and also increased osmosis due to collection of lactic acid, thereby causing flap necrosis by another mechanism.

7. *Free radical formation*—this is primarily superoxide, which is produced by mitochondria as a part of ATP production and other oxidation reduction reactions. Another way in which superoxide radicals are released into the circulation is by white blood cells such as neutrophils, as a direct result of bacterial infection. Free radicals can also be produced in the presence of ischemia by the enzyme xanthine oxidase. This happens when hypoxanthine is produced from high-energy phosphate compounds and accumulates in the tissues. When reperfusion occurs and the partial pressure of oxygen increases in the tissue, the hypoxanthine is converted to uric acid through the action of xanthine oxidase, and this catalytic reaction also causes the production of superoxide as a by-product of the same process. Superoxide causes peroxidation of the lipid layer of the cell membrane and denaturation of the intracellular matrix, thus causing tissue damage. Free radicals can moreover lead to delays in the process of neovascularization and thereby adversely affect endothelial cell proliferation.

8. *Capillary obstruction*—this is due to spasm of the small blood vessels and causes a no-reflow phenomenon in the flap and a high risk of flap necrosis.

The biomechanics of a flap may be influenced by the stress-strain curve. This includes creep which is nothing but the increase in strain that occurs when the skin is subjected to a constant force or stress. Strain is the change in length as compared to the original length. Stress relaxation is the opposite of creep and is the decrease in the forces when a constant strain is used to hold the skin together under tension.

The stress-strain curve can be optimized with the use of flap undermining. This makes use of the shearing force, in other words, the force that is used to neutralize the tension between the dermis and underlying tissue. Reduction in the shearing forces and thereby tension at the edges of a wound has been found in animal studies when the skin edges are undermined up to 4 cm.

The viability and survival of a flap can be enhanced by the following mechanisms:

1. *Increase in the vascular supply*—this may be influenced by factors such as hypotension, infection, or compression of the pedicle of the flap and should therefore be avoided. A technique known as flap delay can be useful and utilizes the staged harvest of a flap to ensure its health and durability.

2. *The use of vasodilators*—these may act indirectly, such as the alpha-adrenergic blocking agents, namely, phenoxybenzamine and phentolamine, or by the depletion of norepinephrine stores, namely reserpine and guanethidine, and anesthetics namely, isoflurane, verapamil and lidocaine, which are better as compared to nitrous oxide for the survival of the flap. Others may have a direct action, and these include histamine, nitroglycerin, nifedipine, hydralazine, pentoxifylline, isoxsuprine, and dimethyl sulfoxide given topically. These may or may not improve flap survival but have not been proven to be harmful.

   Other agents are the calcitonin gene-related peptide (CGRP) which has strong vasodilator action and also encourages the relaxation of smooth muscle, and capsaicin which may be used as a pretreatment. It improves flap viability by depletion of neuropeptides from the primary sensory neurons. Prostaglandins E1 and E2 have proven beneficial in random flaps for reducing skin necrosis.

3. *Neovascularization*—agents such as the vascular endothelial growth factor (VEGF) have been shown to enhance the viability and survival of a flap. Growth factors are especially useful when used for patients who have undergone radiation therapy or suffer from diabetes and steroid dependency which could cause deficiencies in the blood supply.

4. *Rheology*—blood viscosity may be reduced with the use of pentoxifylline and whole blood substitutes. Pentoxifylline acts by interfering with the accumulation of platelets and enhancing the capacity of red blood cells to deform and adjust according to the size of the blood vessel and the capillary circulation pressure, and thus pass easily across tissue interfaces.

5. *Inflammation*—if procedures such as sympathectomy or division of vessels have not been done, then the products of inflammation may be able to improve the viability of the flap. Prostaglandins act by increasing the deformability of red blood cells and decreasing platelet aggregation, thus helping to improve flap survival. Glucocorticoids may be useful as they inhibit phospholipase activity and tissue breakdown. The by-products of the cyclooxygenase pathway, such as COX inhibitors, namely indomethacin and ibuprofen, help to improve flap viability.

6. *A tissue expander*—this provides another useful option. Tissue expanders have also been found to improve the viability and survival of flaps. A tissue expander is a balloon lined with silicon and filled with saline in incremental amounts in order to stretch the skin under which it is inserted. A valve connects the saline chamber to an external site placed at a distant but convenient site so that the saline may be injected into the inner compartment. Fifty to 100 cm^3 of saline may be filled at a time after the initial volume up to a maximum volume of 1000 cm^3. The size of the tissue expander is determined according to the site of the wound, the characteristics of the skin such as elasticity and strength, and the amount of correction required. It is usually kept in situ for 8–12 weeks until the skin has been stretched to the desired capacity and it is possible to suture the skin edges without undue tension. Complications caused by such devices are extrusion, migration, cellulitis, and infection, which would necessitate removal of the same. Tissue expanders are especially useful in the head and neck region when an implant needs to be inserted for a cosmetic or functional purpose. It is crucial

to plan the placement of the implant correctly when it is likely to be in a dependent position such as the neck. In such cases it is useful to tether the implant to the periosteum of the jaw bone to prevent a downward pull on the facial soft tissue and possibly resulting in complications such as ectropion.

7. *Systemic factors*—factors such as tobacco and alcohol use, radiation, or diabetes may influence the behavior of free or vascularized flaps.

Viability of a flap over a period of time can be ensured by:

1. *Protecting it from noxious agents* and introducing a favorable environment, for example, by increasing the concentration of local nitric oxide. The formation of free radicals such as superoxide may lead to the production of hydrogen peroxide by the process of dismutation. Though hydrogen peroxide is not toxic, it may be converted into the more reactive hydroxyl radical. This may be aggravated by the occurrence of a hematoma under the flap. This is due to the breakdown of hemoglobin into iron, which is an important catalyst in the formation of free radicals, and thus the survival of the flap is compromised.

   The use of medicinal leeches or leeching with chemical or mechanical agents, the use of urokinase as an antithrombotic agent, and other techniques, such as extracorporeal circulation, have also been tried and enjoy variable popularity.

2. *Hyperbaric oxygen*—the use of this and also hyperbaric air enhances the oxygen-carrying capacity of the blood by about 20% and thereby the survival of the flap. In addition, it helps to reduce the tendency of the white blood cells to adhere. It also causes vasoconstriction and thus decreases tissue edema and may even be used to salvage a flap. In tissues which have been irradiated, it enhances the process of neovascularization. However, for hyperbaric oxygen to be beneficial, it must be administered early in the treatment, preferably within 24 h of elevation of the flap.

3. *Metabolic manipulation*—this has been tried using agents such as ATP-magnesium chloride complex and difluoromethylornithine in experimental rats and heat-shock proteins in human beings. They are not very popular in use.

3.2 Mechanisms of Injury

3.2.1 Traumatic Brain Injury (TBI)

Traumatic brain injury (TBI) is broadly classified as closed and penetrating head injuries. The 2009 Veterans Administration/Department of Defense clinical practice guidelines (CPGs) are followed in North America. Further classification is done on the basis of signs and symptoms (according to the level of consciousness or sensorium), imaging studies such as CT scan (concussion, contusion, diffuse axonal injury, hematoma, or hemorrhage), anatomic nature (according to the part of the brain involved—subdural hematoma, pontine hemorrhage, and so on), and on the Glasgow Coma Scale or GCS (which also measures the level of consciousness and assigns a score to determine the management protocol).

According to the GCS, a score of 15 with no history of loss of consciousness and no neurological deficit is considered normal or suggestive of minimal injury such as a simple concussion, a score of 14–15 with loss of consciousness of less than 5 min with no neurological impairment is considered mild TBI, and a score of 9–13 with loss of consciousness for more than 5 min with neurological problems is considered moderate, and a score below this is severe head injury, often requiring the airway to be secured with endotracheal intubation.

3.2.2 Source of Injury

3.2.2.1 Blasts and Gunshots

1. *Gunshot*—a detailed discussion of the forensics and technical aspects of missile and gunshot injuries is beyond the purview of this text, but suffice it to say that such matters are extremely crucial when dealing with war wounds and cases of foul play. The make and caliber of the weapon have implications for the kind of injury caused. Devitalization of tissue caused by such injuries, besides causing direct damage, also causes ischemic necrosis of surrounding tissue by vasospasm and the release of toxic chemicals from embedded gunpowder. Blast injuries also have similar effects. The impact of the projectile, for example a bullet, is seen at both the entry and exit points of the projectile. The point of entry is smaller as it goes through clean and healthy tissue. Upon entry into the body, it causes breakdown of deeper tissue and thereafter lacerates or tears through the body to emerge at another point, usually diametrically opposite or in a nonlinear fashion if it is deflected by internal structures. The exit wound is therefore larger and more devitalized and more obvious as a result. Sometimes a patient search must be made for the entry wound as it can be very small or hidden.

2. *Blast and gunshot injuries* cause trauma at more than one level and may be divided into the following:

   (a) *Primary*—direct impact, effect, and interaction with the body tissue.

   (b) *Secondary*—energized particles or projectiles traveling at high speed, which are capable of causing collateral damage by getting deflected or disintegrated upon the primary victim or other persons in the nearby vicinity.

   (c) *Tertiary*—the impact of the projectile may cause actual physical displacement of the victim and as a result expose the individual to other potential sources of trauma, for example a person shot in the chest may fall some distance away, thus sustaining head and neck injuries.

   (d) *Quaternary*—collateral damage such as the glare of the explosion causing blindness and ocular damage, acoustic trauma causing hearing loss, thermal and chemical burns due to heated shrapnel and toxic substances released by embedded particles, and last but not least, psychological trauma not only due to the circumstances of the primary injury but also the period thereafter. This last aspect, referred to as post-traumatic stress disorder (PTSD), is sometimes underdiagnosed and suboptimally treated, leading to serious problems with the rehabilitation process.

3.2.2.2 Burns

A lot of traumatic events are due to burns, and these form a special group. Burns may occur as solitary injuries or be part of the primary trauma. For example, many motor vehicle accidents are due to mechanical trauma from solid objects and also thermal and chemical injuries in the form of burns, such as fire or steam escaping from the engine or noxious substances from the exhaust pipes. Burns are classified into three kinds in terms of severity. First-degree burns refer to those that are limited to the epidermis. Pain is severe in this type of burns, and so is the fluid loss, giving rise to the term "burn shock" or a state of hypovolemia brought about by the rapid loss of water from the tissues in extreme cases. As the dermis and adnexal structures are spared, the reparation process restores complete integrity to the skin over a period of time when full healing has occurred.

Second-degree burns are also known as partial thickness burns and involve the skin and underlying dermis with its adnexal structures. Thus, along with the twin problems of severe pain and burn shock, poor scars are likely to form due to the deposition of large amounts of fibrous tissue which undergoes contraction. Such contractures can cause serious external deformity because the healing is mainly due to secondary intention as primary closure is not possible due to extensive loss of tissue. Large tracts of skin and adnexa are therefore left to heal and contract on their own and the only resort would be to correct these using skin grafts.

Third-degree burns traverse the entire thickness of the skin, even up to the point where bone may be exposed. In other words, they destroy the skin and all of the adnexa with its glands, vessels, muscles, and nerves and are thus not accompanied by pain, though the loss of fluid can be considerable and often fatal. As may be expected, no regeneration of the skin or underlying tissue can occur, and the part may have to be sacrificed or repaired using prosthetic appliances in order to restore a cosmetically acceptable appearance. However, primary reconstruction in such cases is not advisable, and at least 6 months should be allowed for the scar or wound to undergo maturation, and any acute medical or surgical condition must be addressed in order to achieve a stable course. Local dressings with the application of silver sulfadiazine help to prevent infection in burn wounds and minimize further loss of fluids. This is the optimal treatment for extensive burns and may have to be carried out for weeks or months. After this, repair and reconstruction may be undertaken.

3.2.2.3 Radiation-Induced Injury

Radiation-induced injury is similar to burn injury and may be classified into four grades:

(a) *Erythema or mild inflammation.*
(b) *Erythema and discoloration* with dry desquamation (the outermost layer of the epithelium is separated from the deeper layers).
(c) *Inflammation and edema* with wet desquamation—the deeper layers of the epithelium are also separated, along with cell death and loss of fluid from the extracellular compartment.

(d) *Ulceration*—full thickness loss of tissue in the epithelium or deeper layers of the skin or mucous membrane, with or without bleeding.

3.2.2.4 Lesser Degrees of Soft Tissue Trauma

Lesser degrees of soft tissue trauma may also occur resulting in various degrees of laceration with exposure of underlying cartilage. Primary suturing is possible in most cases after careful inspection, irrigation, and debridement of the wound to remove embedded foreign bodies or dirt and grime. Skin approximation should be paid careful attention to as this is an area of the body where a cosmetic result is of utmost importance. Good suturing principles and practice would ensure a good outcome no matter who the person doing the repair is, in other words, the trainee doctor in ENT, a practicing otolaryngologist, or a specialist plastic and reconstructive surgeon.

When the cartilage is exposed or split, the ends of the wound tend to be further away than in cases where only the skin is injured. This is because of relative rigidity of the cartilage, which tends to splay the wound. In these cases, the ends of the cartilage should be brought as close to each other as possible or even slightly overlapped and sutured together with fine absorbable material so as not to give way. The skin edges are then approximated and sutured together.

3.2.2.5 Frostbite

Frostbite is a type of thermal injury occurring due to extreme cold. It is mainly encountered in high-altitude climbers and adventure sports enthusiasts in areas with a cold climate or in cases of accidental exposure. It thus occurs in persons with inadequate coverage of the exposed parts of the face and is rarely seen in local residents or people native to the region. It is recognized by erythema or redness of the skin along with severe pain and tenderness over the site, as in other kinds of thermal injury. The area then gradually turns darker or lighter depending on how early treatment has been instituted. A darker color implies that the area is turning gangrenous and is potentially serious as it may lead to perichondritis. Treatment is carried out with gradual rewarming at 38–42 °C; no direct heat or cold (ice) is to be applied to discolored or inflamed areas.

In impending or suspected perichondritis, hyperbaric oxygen therapy must be instituted as soon as possible in order to improve outcomes.

3.2.3 Prompt Detection

Prompt detection especially in the case of thermal injury is therefore of utmost importance, and treatment is started immediately by thawing of the site using irrigation with sterile saline at room temperature or a warm padding till the redness subsides and further inflammation is prevented. Antibiotic creams, calamine, or silver sulfadiazine may also be applied, but oral medication apart from the occasional painkiller is usually not required. A soft and gentle dressing may be applied if necessary to prevent further exposure.

3.3   Hemostasis, Anesthesia, and Wound Closure

3.3.1   Maintaining Hemostasis and Homeostasis

Hemorrhage of any kind could be fatal if allowed to continue undetected and unabated for several hours. Most of this would not be obvious hemorrhage, as for example when a person bleeds into the abdominal, thoracic, pelvic, or intracranial cavity. Only external signs and assessment of the general condition and vital parameters of the patient would reveal clues as to the presence of such bleeding. It is not only the loss of blood volume but also developments such as compression by the expanding hematoma, especially inside the skull, and the eventual consumption of coagulation factors leading to a state of disseminated intravascular coagulation or DIC, that may ultimately prove fatal.

The causes of shock following injury include hypovolemia secondary to hemorrhage (most common), cardiogenic or pump failure (cardiac tamponade, tension pneumothorax, or myocardial contusion), neurogenic (often combined with hypovolemic shock and masked), and septic (a late event occurring more than 24 h later and often associated with missed fecal spillage).

The responses to initial fluid challenge include an early and guaranteed return of the normal vital signs, but this may be a transient response and a gradual or rapid worsening of the situation may follow. If there is no improvement, a meticulous secondary survey should follow to reassess the presence of potentially life-threatening injuries such as pulmonary or myocardial contusion, a tear of the aorta, diaphragm, tracheobronchial tree, or esophagus.

3.3.2   Skin Closure

Skin edges must be approximated close together to minimize the chances of cross-hatching and a festering wound infection, which may lead to a depressed scar that renders the outcome of the injury worse than the initial injury. It is good practice to keep in hand a set of fine suturing instruments like forceps and needle holder as is common with many facial plastic surgeons.

Simple methods to remove contaminating debris from wounds are gentle irrigation, controlled suction, scrubbing, and dermabrasion. This is important prior to undertaking repair of the wound in order to reduce the chances of impaction and retention of foreign bodies and bone fragments from the patient's own body in the soft tissues of the wound and surrounding region. If such contamination has been missed in the early stages, vaporization by laser may be utilized for its removal.

Primary repair is usually carried out with the help of local flaps, or the wound is allowed to heal by secondary intention. Full or partial thickness skin grafts are an option, but in the treatment of facial soft tissue trauma, skin grafts may not always provide a good tissue and color match. Scar revision may be undertaken for persistent ugly scars resulting from the initial treatment.

3.3.3   Local Anesthesia

Most soft tissue injuries without serious accompanying trauma may be repaired using a topical anesthetic agent such as TAC (tetracaine, adrenaline, cocaine) or LAT (4% lidocaine, 1:200,000 adrenaline, 1% tetracaine). Lidocaine is eminently suitable as its action is more localized and the systemic toxicity is less. The problem with the use of cocaine is its potential for abuse and relative ease of identification during drug testing. This aspect may be extremely important in professional sportsmen who must be treated for trauma. Children may resist the administration of any kind of treatment including the initial anesthesia, and they must be cleverly distracted, and applicators are used for the local anesthesia. Injection is painful and may be avoided in children. The pain is caused by the acidic pH, which is 4.0, of the anesthetic agent. This is the optimum pH to be maintained as it ensures the hydrostatic and chemical effects of the anesthetic. Buffering with sodium bicarbonate (1 ml 8.4% sodium bicarbonate and 9 ml 1% lidocaine in 1:100,000 adrenaline brings the pH to a more tolerable 7.0 but results in a shorter duration of action lasting for 30–45 min. If the procedure is likely to take more time, sedation or a general anesthetic agent may be used instead.

3.3.4   Suturing Tips

Suture materials must also be chosen with care. Good results are obtained with the use of 7.0 nylon sutures in adults, whereas absorbing gut sutures are best in children. Polyglycolic acid sutures may cause a foreign body reaction as they do not degrade completely. This may result in inflammation and infection, producing a wide and depressed scar which looks unacceptably bad. While approximating the skin edges, care should be taken not to include fat and muscle as these structures provide less tensile strength and may be absorbed over time, especially muscle. Good tension and approximation are provided by fascia and subcutaneous tissues, so these are the layers to be used for suturing. A wide and depressed scar may also be the result of extensive soft tissue contusion with loss of subcutaneous tissue. Hyperbaric oxygen, platelet inhibitors or anticoagulants, and medicinal leeches are useful for reducing venous congestion and improving the viability of soft tissue in severe avulsion injuries.

Special care must be taken while suturing the margins of the wound in areas such as the vermilion border, eyelid, and rim of the nose and helix of the ear. When cleaning the wound near the eye and nose, the lacrimal gland must be protected from injury.

3.3.5   Surgical Outcomes

Trauma such as a pelvic crush injury or limb fracture releases products of muscle breakdown, and these lead to an intense inflammatory response, but both of them individually or together are capable of causing serious injury to the kidneys and an acute renal shutdown. The inability of the kidneys to clear the circulation causes further accumulation of toxins in the body and aggravates the acute kidney injury, causing a vicious cycle. Furthermore, the kidneys are not able to produce erythropoietin when damaged, and this exacerbates the already anemic state that occurs due to the blood loss caused by the traumatic event. This sequence of events could span several days causing a tumultuous progression of the inciting trauma and its aftermath.

Therefore the effect of trauma on the body depends primarily on the cause or mechanism and the time taken to treatment. The cascade of steps or events in this process decides whether the injury is reversible or not, in other words, whether repair, rehabilitation, and a return to normalcy can be expected or a terminal event such as loss of life, limb, or function will occur instead.

Although the head, face, and neck region has a robust vascular supply and healing occurs within as few as 5 days, the potential for infection is also great owing to the rich microbiome that exists in the mucosa-lined cavities of the ear, nose, and throat. Host factors such as poor nutrition, poor immunity, and poor hygiene also contribute to the propensity for wounds in this region to get infected. Such infections pose a tremendous risk to the intracranial cavity as well as the systemic circulation and hence must be prevented and treated aggressively. Good surgical technique, thorough cleansing of wounds, adequate antibiotic cover, and attention to health and hygiene should be sufficient measures for the prevention of infection. The use of prophylactic antibiotics for faciomaxillary trauma is generally not recommended because the face has a rich arterial blood supply and an efficient venous drainage. Thus even though resident microflora abound on the mucosal surfaces and in the lymphoid tissues of the face, infection is not really a threat. Antibiotics may be reserved for patients with known risk factors such as diabetes and other causes of immunosuppression and confounding factors for the wound such as the presence of animal bites and wound contamination [5].

In the event that the wound gets infected though, sutures if any must be removed at once, the wound debrided and cleaned, and either healing by secondary intention may be allowed or secondary suturing done if adequate margins remain after the debridement. Such wounds may be left open most of the time and signs of cellulitis, cavernous sinus thrombosis, meningitis and encephalitis, and neck space infections watched for.

3.3.6 Adjuvant Treatment

Tetanus prophylaxis may be given in the case of contaminated wounds or in cases where the nature of environmental factors at the time of injury is not known. It is also given when the patient has not taken tetanus immunization according to the schedule pertaining to that region.

3.4   Optimizing Management

Trauma constitutes one of the commonest causes of mortality and morbidity all over the world, closely following cardiovascular and lifestyle diseases, cancer, and infection. It is not difficult to understand why. With the rise in urbanization, conflict, and strife, trauma could easily take center stage, and the various modes by which it could affect human populations are physical violence, motor vehicle or road traffic accidents, accidental falls, child and elder abuse, and other causes such as contact sports and adventure or extreme sports. Added to this litany would be iatrogenic trauma, which is coming more and more into the forefront as instances of medical error, due not only to the increased accessibility to medical services but also the complex mechanisms by which medical care is delivered.

Complex trauma is best managed in a dedicated trauma center. Smaller establishments are only equipped to provide first aid. They also serve to stabilize the patient till adequate and safe transportation to a referral center can be provided. Trauma centers function on the basis of optimal infrastructure and the presence of active multidisciplinary teams, with a well-oiled machinery to follow trauma protocols and the capacity for sound decision making at all levels of management. In any other kind of setup, the usual problems arise as a result of clashes among various specialists looking after the trauma survivor. Lack of communication and coordination may lead to delays, complications, and suboptimal treatment.

As head and neck trauma is seriously life threatening and involves vital structures such as the brain and cerebral circulation, the airway and the organs of special sense, circulation, and breathing must be established first and foremost. The ENT surgeon is fast emerging as the hero in the acute management of trauma especially because of mastery over handling the airway, ability to tackle major bleeding in the head and neck region, and the endoscopic skills required for detecting injury to internal structures and organs.

The MTOS (*major trauma outcome study*) is useful for the measurement of the severity of injury and to systematically document management and outcomes for future reference and periodic audit and to provide a roadmap for evaluating performance and quality of care.

The effect of trauma may be major or lethal, as when it causes death or a terminal event such as permanent loss of function. The extent to which trauma could affect human physiology mainly depends on what function is compromised first. If the airway is involved as in obstruction or pneumothorax, or brainstem injury paralyzing the respiratory center, death could ensue rapidly in a matter of seconds to minutes. Many such cases would not make it to a medical facility in time but much depends on the availability of trauma services pertaining to that region.

The management of trauma has undergone a radical change over the last few decades. While the mortality and morbidity from trauma was high in earlier times when the time taken for the patient to reach a medical aid facility was the chief limiting factor, the advent of critical care services and life support systems have ensured that a trauma patient can be potentially salvaged if at all brought to a hospital in a live condition. However, saving a life is not the end of the story. Modern medicine is capable of maintaining life in the most adverse circumstances with the aid of machines and monitors. This brings into the picture all the other processes that go wrong while trying to achieve this. A body crushed and mangled beyond reasonable capacity to sustain itself is still technically alive because of medications, mechanical ventilation, and a myriad of other interventions that help in the continuation of cellular activities. There is a pulse, blood pressure, respiratory rate, and body temperature that proclaim that a person is still alive. What it fails to take into account is that all these would cease to exist if any of the external factors is removed, in other words, death would ensue without the use of life support equipment. But it would be futile to argue this. Medicine is always hopeful, and thus the life of a man (or woman) must be preserved at any cost whatsoever, by natural means or artificial. One would not wish to think otherwise.

It is therefore worthwhile considering what actually happens during the preservation of life of a trauma victim. Much depends on the age, nature of trauma, and timely medical help. Each kind of trauma taken individually places a different degree of stress on the body. A patient with head injury is the most vulnerable because the respiratory system could shut down rapidly and result in death. Thus if artificial ventilation is instituted in time, the patient lives. The site and extent of the head injury then determines the further prognosis. A concussion injury to the brain has a good outcome, while a diffuse axonal injury does not. A localized extradural hematoma or limited subarachnoid hemorrhage carries a better prognosis than an extensive subdural hematoma or hemorrhage in the brainstem.

Next in terms of seriousness is abdominal and thoracic cage trauma. Abdominal trauma could be lethal on account of blood loss but takes more time to evolve thus giving doctors a chance to help the patient. Pneumothorax due to trauma to the chest and resulting in rib fracture(s), however, can be acutely life threatening and needs to be managed expediently, perhaps only a tad less aggressively than managing head injury. In this case, not only does the airway need to be secured but an intercostal drain also needs to be inserted quickly before even mechanical ventilation can be carried out.

Pelvic and long limb trauma come a close second to head, abdominal, or chest trauma. Both result in severe crush injuries and release of products of muscle and tissue breakdown, inflammatory mediators, and air or fat embolism. These may cause an acute kidney shutdown or aggravate a pre-existing renal compromise due to age, pre-existing hypertension, or diabetes mellitus. Acute kidney injury means that much of the blood loss resulting from the trauma cannot be made up to the desired extent and with the requisite urgency. Any kind of blood product—whole blood, platelets, or plasma—cannot be given freely as this could cause worsening of the stress on the kidneys. Heme production is also brought to a standstill as the production of renal erythropoietin by the body is affected as well.

Gradual deterioration in the patient's condition ensues as the vital parameters worsen due to continuing blood loss, inability to intervene surgically or aggressively in view of the poor renal status, progressive release of the mediators of inflammation, and eventually the most dreaded complication of all—DIC or disseminated intravascular coagulation—that finally spells the death knell for the patient. In all this time, nevertheless, the patient has been maintained on artificial life support. Even if he or she survives miraculously, a return to normalcy or near normalcy would be difficult to expect, bringing forth serious questions about the utility of modern methods of trauma management or, to be more precise, their futility in being able to deliver scientifically optimal, socially rational, and cost-effective outcomes.

A provision for special needs adds to the quality of care for trauma survivors. Metabolic beds, water and air beds, ventilators with customizable adjustments, and so on may be required for certain patients who have complications or comorbid conditions. Patients with pre-existing illness must have proper guidance and counseling once the acute management is over and discharge from the hospital planned. For example, an obese patient with untreated or undiagnosed sleep apnea may suffer trauma and be in hospital for a variable period of time, getting a tracheotomy for airway management, which by default serves to ameliorate the symptoms of sleep apnea as well. At the time of discharge, the tracheotomy may be removed without concern for the underlying sleep apnea. Such a patient may be at grave risk of serious morbidity and mortality in the period of convalescence. Such special situations need to be examined closely and the patient advised to either continue with the tracheotomy or other modes of home therapy must be applied. These include the use of a CPAP (continuous positive airway pressure) or BiPAP (bi-level or biphasic positive airway pressure).

In many instances, the primary trauma is dealt with fairly satisfactorily, but all the interventions put together mean a terribly prolonged hospital stay, a severe drain on resources, and a host of iatrogenic complications and suboptimal rehabilitation, preventing a restoration to normal conditions. For example, airway intervention through intubation or tracheotomy might result in airway stenosis, which may be missed or misdiagnosed in the rehabilitation of the primary trauma, and thus prevent decanulation and a return to normalcy.

Timing of definitive surgery after trauma is an important concern where trauma complicates a pre-existing condition. For instance, a tympanic membrane perforation or a deviated nasal septum may be neglected by the patient for a long time until there is an episode of trauma to the head and neck. Injury to the external ear or temporal bone, or to the nasal bones and facial skeleton, may aggravate the otherwise insidious progression of a conductive hearing loss or nasal obstruction. It is crucial to determine the optimal timing for surgical intervention in such a situation, and this would obviously depend on individual needs and constraints.

Post-traumatic stress disorder (PTSD), the more commonly known name for trauma-related stress, is one of the least discussed issues in trauma practice. It may follow minor or major trauma, more often the latter, and is more likely to be encountered in sensitive yet strong individuals, especially those with relatively less social or family support in the aftermath of the trauma. An introverted, diffident, or pessimistic disposition may also contribute, and this condition is further complicated by financial or legal hassles in getting satisfactory treatment for the injury, including the process of rehabilitation.

Anxiety, depression, insomnia, irritability, panic attacks, violence, and the unmasking of a bipolar disorder are the usual ways in which PTSD may manifest itself and interfere with the overall management of the traumatic event.

Psychological problems may also be seen in cases of domestic or spousal abuse, in which the suffering party may actually try to cover up the details and present with suspicious, extraordinary, or dramatic complaints. It takes an astute clinician to sniff out the truth and take the treatment along a medically and ethically sound course.

Trauma to the soft tissues of face is fairly common as the face is in an extremely vulnerable position being directly exposed to the external environment. Thus the effects of such trauma are not only physical but also cause an immense impact on the emotional, psychological, and social aspects as well. It is vital to rule out abuse in children, women, and elderly persons.

Counseling of the patient, reassurance for the patient and family, professional care, and the remediation of social, ethical, or legal issues are as important as the medical or surgical treatment of the physical wounds of the injurious event.

The important aspects of wound healing and trauma care are summarized in Table 3.1.

Table 3.1 Determinants of wound healing in a nutshell

Aspects of wound healing						
Zones of blood flow	Modes of injury	Common causes of shock	Crucial factors	Types of flaps	Major factors in flap	Other factors in flap
	Gunshot	Blood loss	Complex trauma	Random cutaneous	Blood supply	Infection
1. Systemic circulation	Blast	Heart failure	Prognosis	Arterial cutaneous	Micro circulation	Reperfusion
2. Capillary circulation	Burns	Tension pneumo thorax	Special needs	Myo cutaneous	New vessel formation	Free radical formation
3. Interstitial spaces	Radiation	Neurogenic	Timing of surgery	Free micro vascular	Nerve section	Capillary obstruction
4. Cells and membranes	Frostbite	Septic	PTSD			

Conclusion

A sound knowledge and understanding of trauma at the tissue level must be combined with the technical aspects such as the mechanisms of injury. Attention to hemostasis and homeostasis, anesthesia, and suturing techniques is a crucial determinant in the optimal management of trauma.

References

1. Sidle DM, Decker JR. Use of makeup, hairstyles, glasses, and prosthetics as adjuncts to scar camouflage. Facial Plast Surg Clin North Am. 2011;19(3):481–9
2. Shockley WW. Scar revision techniques. Oper Tech Otolaryngol Head Neck Surg. 2011;22(1):84–93
3. Christophel JJ, Elm C, Endrizzi BT, Hilger PA, Zelickson B. A randomized controlled trial of fractional laser therapy and dermabrasion for scar resurfacing. Dermatol Surg. 2012;38(4):595–602
4. Thomas JR, Somenek M. Scar revision review. Arch Facial Plast Surg. 2012;14(3):162–74
5. Abubaker AO. Use of prophylactic antibiotics in preventing infection of traumatic injuries. Oral Maxillofac Surg Clin North Am. 2009;21(2):259–64. vii

Learning Objectives
- To learn the pathophysiology of trauma to the ear
- To understand the clinical implications of management of ear trauma
- To remember the best practice recommendations in ear trauma

4.1   Pathophysiology

4.1.1   Embryology and Applied Anatomy

At about 22 days, when the embryo is at the 7-somite stage, the primitive ear is formed as the otic placode. At 30 days and 3-somite stage, the otocyst has formed which goes on enlarging and differentiating. The outer ear is first evident at 8 weeks and achieves adult form by 16 weeks though further enlargement continues thereafter till birth and then up to adulthood. Though the middle ear cleft is fully formed by 8 months of intrauterine life, the air cells are still filled with amniotic fluid, which gets replaced by air soon after birth. The middle ear ossicles—malleus, incus, and stapes—are fully formed by 25 weeks. By 21 weeks, the otic capsule completes its ossification from 14 centers and attains the adult size, and at 25 weeks, the definitive inner ear with specialized neuroepithelium and adult structure has been formed.

4.1.2   The Outer Ear

The outer ear is composed of the pinna or auricle, the external or outer ear canal, and the external layer of the eardrum or tympanic membrane. The pinna has two portions, the upper cartilaginous part composed of yellow elastic cartilage covered by skin, which gives form and shape to the ear, and the lower fatty portion called lobule which is adipose tissue covered with skin. The outer epidermal layer of the tympanic membrane migrates at the rate of 0.05 mm per day, and this roughly denotes the time taken for a perforation to heal spontaneously.

The outer ear or auricle receives sensory supply from five nerves. The principal sensory nerve is the greater auricular, formed by the cervical nerves 2 and 3, and this supplies sensation to the medial surface and also the lateral surface toward its posterior half. The lesser occipital derived from the second cervical nerve supplies the medial surface on its upper portion. The auriculotemporal nerve derived from the mandibular branch of the fifth or trigeminal nerve supplies the tragus and part of helix. A twig from the vagus or tenth cranial nerve supplies the concha, eminentia conchae, and antihelix. This nerve is called Arnold's nerve, and it may get stimulated while syringing the ear for the removal of wax or foreign bodies, triggering the cough reflex, or in severe cases, a syncopal attack. A branch from the facial nerve supplies a very small region at the root of the concha.

While administering local anesthesia to the ear, the sensory innervations of the outer ear must be borne in mind. Most surgical procedures including those for the treatment of trauma may be carried out by infiltrating the points of entry of the above nerves.

4.1.3 Barotrauma

Barotrauma is known by synonyms such as aviation pressure deafness and aero-otitis media, and anecdotal evidence can be found on the description of this entity as recorded by Sydney Scott during the First World War. He outlined the precautions and care to be taken by pilots in order to avoid barotrauma. It was also a common occurrence in the Second World War thanks to the widespread use of airborne forces. It may be easily explained on the basis of Boyle's Law, which states that pressure is inversely proportional to volume in a fixed mass of gas. In practical terms, the environmental pressure decreases as altitude increases. It is half of the normal atmospheric pressure at 18,000 ft and only a quarter at 34,000 ft. There is an increase of 1 atmosphere pressure with every 10 m underwater. If the pressure gradient increases more than 90 mm of mercury, the auditory tube gets locked. The middle ear is now not able to equilibrate air pressure and barotrauma occurs. It is caused by pressure disequilibrium across the tympanic membrane when the Eustachian tube fails to ventilate the ear. This usually happens in case of excessive increase in middle ear pressure beyond a certain point when the Eustachian tube is normal and also in a sudden increase in volume of the middle ear space when the tube is malfunctioning. Rapid ascent or descent, nasal infections, polyps, or allergy may precipitate barotraumas. Infants and young children also suffer more from barotrauma because of the shorter, wider, straighter, and immature auditory tube in comparison with adults.

Barotrauma to the ear may occur by several mechanisms. Normally the Eustachian or auditory tube passively allows air to escape from the middle ear cleft in order to equalize middle ear pressure. This is necessary when the external or atmospheric pressure falls, and consequently the middle ear volume rises while pressure falls. This happens during the ascent stage of a flight or deep sea dive. The increased volume of air in the middle ear cavity would cause passive opening of the auditory tube. If the nasopharyngeal end of the tube is malfunctioning either due to edema or compression from adenoids or nasopharyngeal masses, the tube fails to open passively. The middle ear pressure continues to fall, and a vacuum is created in the middle ear cleft, causing capillaries to rupture and bleed and resulting in effusion or hemotympanum. The patient experiences pain, fullness or ear block, and hearing impairment until the time the insult passes, and the fluid contents are slowly resorbed. Long-term sequelae could be fibrosis, ankylosis, tympanosclerosis, or cholesterol granuloma, all resulting in conductive deafness.

When the atmospheric pressure rises, as happens during the descent phase of a flight or deep sea dive, the middle ear is compressed, and the volume in the middle ear cleft falls, while the pressure rises. This would normally prevent the nasopharyngeal end of the tube from opening passively, and now active muscular action at this end causes the tube to open widely and equalize the middle ear pressure. Active muscular action is brought about and augmented by yawning, swallowing, sucking, and the Toynbee, Muller, and Valsalva maneuvers. All these may be difficult to perform in the event of an upper respiratory tract infection or external compression by adenoids or other masses. The continued rise in pressure leads to capillary hemorrhages and sometimes perforation of the eardrum, resulting in pain and conductive hearing loss.

4.1.4 The Facial Nerve

The facial nerve arises from its nucleus in the midportion of the pons, then traverses the pons to wind around the abducens nerve nucleus on the dorsal aspect of the pons, forming the facial colliculus, and then remerges from the ventral aspect of the pons into the cerebellopontine (CP) angle. Thereafter it enters the fundus of the internal auditory meatus (IAM) and travels in the anterosuperior compartment of the internal auditory canal (IAC) in front of the superior vestibular nerve and above the cochlear nerve to reach the porus of the IAC, at which point it enters the middle ear cavity. This part of the facial nerve is known as the labyrinthine segment. The facial canal is narrowest at its labyrinthine portion where the facial nerve enters the internal acoustic meatus. It measures about 0.7 mm, and therefore the facial nerve in this portion is extremely vulnerable to any kind of edema or compression following trauma or inflammation. The covering of the pia-arachnoid also ends at the fundus of the internal auditory meatus (IAM), forming a tight band across the facial nerve at this point. The labyrinthine artery supplying this segment is a tenuous end artery. These two latter problems add to the propensity of the facial nerve to undergo ischemic injury in this portion.

The facial nerve then turns backward sharply behind the processus cochleariformis, forming the first genu and continuing as the horizontal or tympanic segment until it turns downward at the level of the pyramidal eminence, forming the second genu and continuing as the vertical/longitudinal or mastoid segment, to finally escape from the skull base through the stylomastoid foramen. It then enters the parotid gland to divide into the five terminal branches—temporal, zygomatic, buccal, mandibular, and cervical—at the posterior border of the parotid gland in a formation known as the pes anserinus or the foot of a duck.

The facial nerve nucleus at the pons receives the majority of its innervation from the opposite cerebral cortex, with only the portion for the temporal branch receiving ipsilateral innervations as well. Thus it is that supranuclear lesions spare the upper part of the contralateral but affected side, whereas infranuclear or lower motor neuron lesions cause a complete paralysis of the same side of the face.

From the first genu, the facial nerve gives off the greater superficial petrosal nerve (GSPN). This, together with the deep petrosal nerve derived from the branches of the cervical sympathetic plexus, forms the nerve of the pterygoid canal, otherwise known as the Vidian nerve. It supplies the secretomotor glands of the lacrimal and nasal regions and may be affected in transverse fractures of the temporal bone where the nerve gets sheared at its point of exit from the first genu. Just after the second genu, the facial nerve gives off its nerve to the stapedius which controls the stapedial reflex and then the chorda tympani nerve which is responsible for the perception of taste in the anterior two thirds of the ipsilateral tongue. Both these branches may be injured in transverse fractures of the temporal bone with or without involvement of the otic capsule. The mastoid and subsequent portions of the facial nerve carry motor innervations to the muscles of the face, and injury in these regions could occur from both temporal bone fractures and penetrating injuries of the upper neck region.

The most common manifestation of facial nerve injury is paralysis, and this has been classified by Seddon into three types—neuropraxia, axonotmesis, neurotmesis—and by Sunderland into five types: neuropraxia, axonotmesis, neurotmesis, partial transection (perineural disruption), and complete transection (epineural disruption). The classification system of House and Brackmann is slightly different and is composed of six grades that take into account the muscle groups involved, the functional impairment, and also the nature of return of spontaneous facial nerve activity. The practical aspect of this second classification system is that grade 4 and higher means incomplete eye closure with maximal effort and therefore demands utmost attention to care of the affected eye. Grade 3 paralyses may also necessitate some form of eye care as complete closure takes place only with maximal effort. Grades 5 and 6 of the House-Brackmann classification describe the effects of faulty regeneration of the nerve and the presence of abnormal features such as synkinesia and mass movements.

Facial nerve injury poses three principal problems—eye and corneal exposure with the risk of blindness, inability to express smile and other emotions, and asymmetry of the face at rest leading to a socially frightening and unacceptable appearance. The symptoms produced would be dry eye with epiphora, alteration in taste, hyperacusis and intolerance to sound, as well as weakness of the facial musculature on the affected side.

The facial nerve may be injured in blunt trauma as in temporal bone fractures and penetrating trauma as in physical assault or gunshot injuries, which may injure any portion of the nerve. A third category, caused by human or animal bites, usually involves the extracranial portion of the cranial nerve and may additionally cause injuries over the face and parotid gland.

The facial nerve can also be affected in barotraumas of the ear and result in facial nerve paralysis. This usually occurs when there are natural dehiscences of the facial nerve canal or when the facial canal has been involved in temporal bone trauma. Transmission of pressure waves may then lead to concussion, edema, or inflammation of the exposed facial nerve and cause a facial nerve paresis or palsy depending on the extent of the underlying defect and superimposed injury. This kind of facial weakness is usually temporary and responds to conservative measures. Surgical exploration may be needed when medical or conservative measures fail and would follow the same protocol as that for facial nerve injury seen in temporal bone trauma.

4.1.5 Iatrogenic Trauma

Iatrogenic trauma to the facial nerve is not uncommon and is a painful part of the learning curve of any ENT surgeon. Indeed, popular anecdotes abound as to the proficiency of the otologist who causes a facial nerve paralysis, and that one has not done a good mastoidectomy if one has not injured the facial nerve in the process! In the current era, however, such humor may well be considered to be in extremely bad taste, what with exacting standards for resident training, sophisticated imaging techniques, and the use of intraoperative facial nerve monitoring.

Any trauma, including iatrogenic facial nerve trauma, is most commonly encountered in the tympanic segment because of the considerably high incidence of facial nerve canal dehiscence involving this portion, in roughly 50% of the general population. Causes of facial palsy of immediate onset following temporal bone fracture include nerve transection or laceration, bony spicules and fragments of the facial canal impinging on the nerve, and hematoma(s) compressing the nerve sheath exposed by the injury or in cases of congenital dehiscence.

4.1.6 The Temporal Bone

The temporal bone articulates with the parietal bone above, the sphenoid in front, and the occipital below and behind. It has five parts, namely the squamous, petrous, mastoid, tympanic, and zygomatic, which articulates with the zygoma or cheek bone. The zygomatic process of the temporal bone divides the lateral surface of the skull into the temporal part above and the infratemporal fossa below, which also forms the roof of the glenoid fossa of the temporomandibular joint.

Temporal bone fractures are a kind of skull base fractures, which occur as result of transmission of forces across the suture lines and foramina of the skull base.

These structures are the inherent points of weakness in the skull base, and fracture lines tend to assume typical patterns based on their distribution.

Temporal bone fractures are the result of complex trauma to the head and facial skeleton and thus accompany head injuries and facial fractures, more commonly the former. Though the petrous part of the temporal bone is one of the strongest bones in the body, it is vulnerable to fracture along lines of weakness owing to the shearing forces distributed along the base of the skull. Thus the temporal bone may break at any of its parts—squamous, mastoid, petrous, tympanic ring, or zygomatic process, or even at the styloid process. Along with bone, soft tissue injury also occurs, and neural and vascular elements are also affected.

Temporal bone fractures have traditionally been divided into two broad categories—longitudinal and transverse. Longitudinal fractures are more common and comprise about 80% of fractures, and the rest are transverse fractures. About 25% of longitudinal fractures are seen on both sides. A longitudinal fracture is so called because it occurs along the long axis of the temporal bone—from the external auditory meatus to the apex of the petrous part—and usually traverses the middle ear cleft and auditory tube. It is caused by a lateral impact upon the skull due to direct physical assault with a blunt object, falls to the side, and motor vehicle accidents with a lateral shearing force. It tends to cause more soft tissue than bony injury, and thus external ear abrasions, contusions, or lacerations may be seen. The external auditory canal and the contiguous tympanic membrane may be lacerated or avulsed, and perforations may be seen. Hemotympanum or the presence of blood behind an intact tympanic membrane is common due to bleeding into the middle ear cleft. Pain, bleeding from ear or nose (through the auditory tube), deformity, and conductive hearing loss are seen.

A temporary conductive loss occurs due to the presence of blood or CSF, and this may be left to resolve on its own while watching out for infection. Permanent conductive loss occurs due to incudostapedial joint subluxation or disarticulation, dislocation of the incus, stapes arch fractures, malleus fracture, and finally fixation of the incus or head of the malleus as the outer attic wall is pushed medially or laterally by compressive forces. The injuries listed above occur in the given order of frequency. Although these latter varieties form a severe type of conductive hearing loss, it is not truly permanent in nature as surgical correction may be undertaken if the cochlear reserve is good. A fracture line passing through the Eustachian tube may result in refractory otitis media with effusion due to damage to the Eustachian cushion and would have to be treated with myringotomy and insertion of a ventilation tube.

A transverse fracture refers to the occurrence of the fracture line through the broad aspect of the petrous temporal, thus cutting across it transversely instead of along it longitudinally. The most common site is across the otic capsule—either just in front of it (medial) or behind it (lateral). Thus, it has a high predilection for causing injury to the inner ear and facial nerve. Therefore, even though transverse fractures comprise about 20% of temporal bone fractures, nearly 50% of this type of fracture can cause facial nerve paralysis. Irreversible hearing loss due to damage to the cochlea, or occurrence of a perilymphatic fistula, intractable vertigo, and cerebrospinal fluid (CSF) leak with its attendant morbidity are other features seen with a transverse fracture. Battle's sign or contusion over the mastoid process is considered to be pathognomonic of such a fracture, and the diagnosis is made using imaging with a plain CT brain with temporal cuts or a high-resolution CT (HRCT) temporal bone with 0.8–1 mm cuts in the axial and coronal planes. HRCT is especially helpful when facial paralysis, ossicular discontinuity, CSF leak, or perilymph fistula is present or suspected, in order to guide further investigations and treatment. CSF leak is described in detail in Chap. 5.

A transverse fracture follows a linear path from the foramen magnum to the foramen spinosum across the foramen lacerum, also traversing and affecting on its way the jugular foramen, hypoglossal foramen, and internal auditory meatus. A longitudinal fracture is roughly perpendicular to this, that is, it extends across the squamous part of the temporal bone to the foramen spinosum, passing on its way the posterior superior part of the external auditory canal, upper portion of the middle ear, and the carotid canal. The relative incidences of longitudinal and transverse fractures mentioned above, though the most often cited, are not constant and vary rather widely across the published literature on this topic. Because it is rare to encounter a classic longitudinal or transverse fracture and the fracture line is many a time oblique in course, newer classification systems have evolved and resulted into the terminology of otic capsule sparing (OCS) and otic capsule violating (OCV) types of fracture. OCS is lateral and OCV is medial to the otic capsule. This is a more practical classification, and features of both transverse and longitudinal fractures are seen.

Diagnosis and treatment are therefore need based. Temporal bone fractures in children may have a similar presentation as in adults but with less morbidity as the pneumatization of the mastoid air cells lends a good amount of elasticity and shock-absorbing capacity to the temporal bone and the involved structures.

Diagnosis is made on the basis of history and physical examination, EUM (examination under microscope), audiometry, and imaging with CT scan. Treatment depends on the extent of injury. Soft tissue injuries may be cleaned, sutured, and dressed. Ear canal lacerations if circumferential need to be gently packed with a steroid antibiotic ointment to minimize chances of stenosis, whereas isolated areas of injury may be left to heal on their own without packing, taking care only to maintain aseptic conditions, or prophylactic antibiotics orally if required. Presence of a hemotympanum does not always mean active intervention, aspiration, or drainage, but a strict vigil must be maintained to promptly detect and treat ossicular chain damage or fibrosis.

Blast trauma is due to the transmission of a very strong pressure wave across all the components of the ear—external, middle, and inner. It may be due to an excessively loud noise or an explosive force as is seen in bomb blasts, gunshot, and other ballistic wounds. While loud noise spares the external ear and tends to damage the more delicate middle and inner ear structures, explosions could damage all the three components as they also carry physical particles such as shrapnel and gunpowder and also chemicals or toxins. External ear lacerations, perichondritis, eardrum perforations, ossicular damage, and inner ear barotrauma can also occur. In addition, the spiral lamina of the cochlea may be disrupted leading to various degrees of hearing loss which is usually permanent.

4.2   Clinical Implications

4.2.1   Outer Ear

Earrings and studs are commonly worn over the pinna as cosmetic accessories. They may be pierced into the tissue or attached with a press-style clamp or have a combination of both. Piercing methods may not always be aseptic in nature, and infections are very common and in some cases may lead to serious problems such as perichondritis. Ear manipulation with buds and other solid objects such as hairpins and safety pins is very common and can cause direct trauma to the skin of the ear canal and may even perforate the tympanic membrane if forcibly introduced deeper into the ear, such as when another person pushes or brushes against the user. Medication abuse or routine use of potentially ototoxic eardrops may be considered a form of trauma—both self-induced and iatrogenic. Medication abuse with antibiotic eardrops may lead to fungal infections of the ear canal, while ototoxic medications may cause hearing impairment.

External ear trauma has been classified by Weerda [1] into the following four types:

1. *Minor abrasion*—this type, as the definition suggests, involves minimal intervention in the form of an antibiotic cream for superficial abrasion and primary suturing of the wound with topical or oral antibiotic cover.
2. *Minor avulsion*—where only a part of the pinna has been avulsed but has a pedicle about 5 mm in size with a feeding vessel, primary suturing may be done with fine nonabsorbable monofilament material, taking care to approximate the edges carefully. Oral or topical antibiotic may be prescribed as necessary (Figs. 4.1, 4.2, 4.3, 4.4).

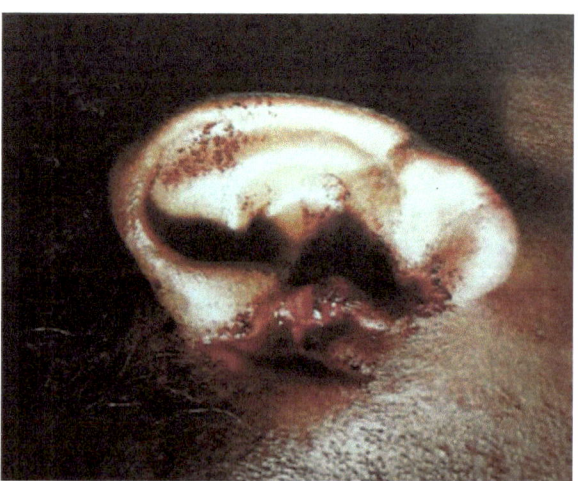

Fig. 4.1 Minor avulsion of pinna

Fig. 4.2 Primary repair of avulsion

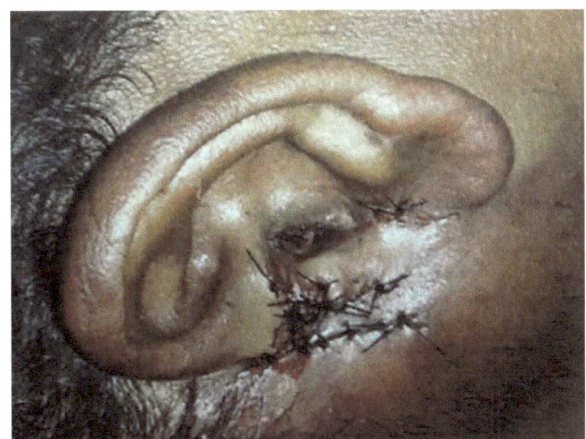

Fig. 4.3 Minor avulsion auricle

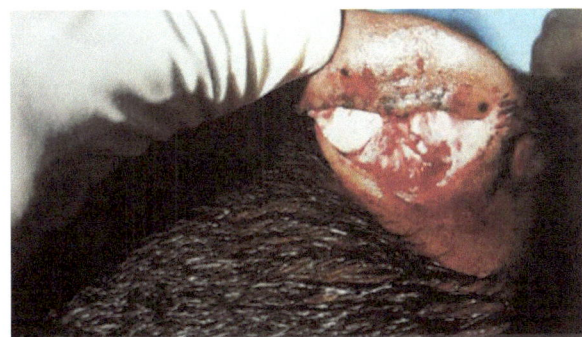

Fig. 4.4 Primary repair avulsion

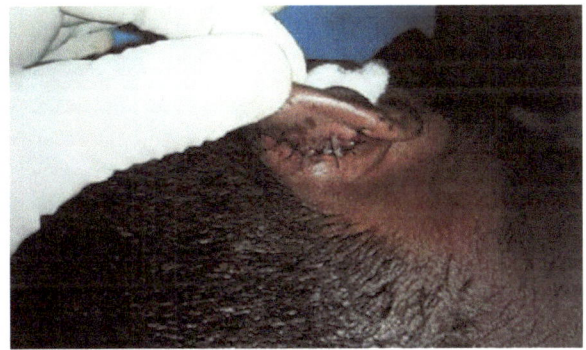

3. *Major avulsion*—if the pinna is avulsed and a large piece up to several millimeters in size is lost or devitalized, the missing part may be sacrificed and primary suturing is still possible. This may be facilitated by undermining the skin edges of the remaining wound. In some areas of the pinna, some distortion of normal anatomy may be acceptable, as over the lobule or rim. The pinna may look

slightly smaller in size as compared to the unaffected side but structurally similar and hence cosmetically all right (Figs. 4.5, 4.6, 4.7, 4.8, 4.9, 4.10).

Primary repair and direct reattachment of an avulsed auricle as a composite graft can be done if the size of the amputated part is smaller than 15 mm in diameter [2].

Even if the amputated segment has suffered an ischemia time of the usual 4–6 h, it does not affect the chances of graft uptake or failure of a directly replanted composite graft, especially if a microsurgical replantation has been carried out [3].

Another method of primary repair is by repositioning the cartilage and covering it with local skin flaps such as a platysma or temporoparietal fascia flap [4]. Salvage surgery as such as Baudet's technique may be utilized if microsurgical replantation is not possible [5]. Baudet's technique is classically described for near total avulsion of the pinna of the auricle following animal or human bite and involves tucking of the amputated stump in the retroauricular sulcus, providing an acceptable cosmetic appearance [6].

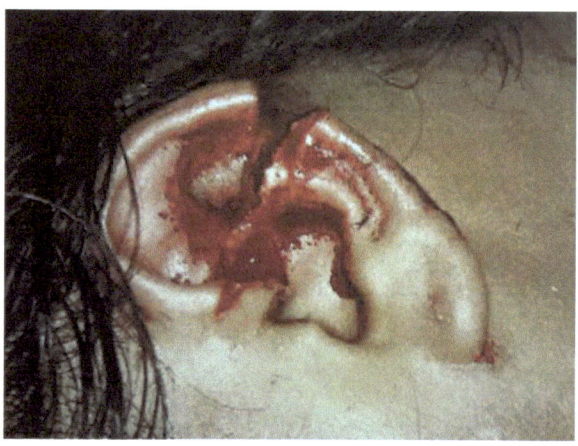

Fig. 4.5 Major avulsion of pinna

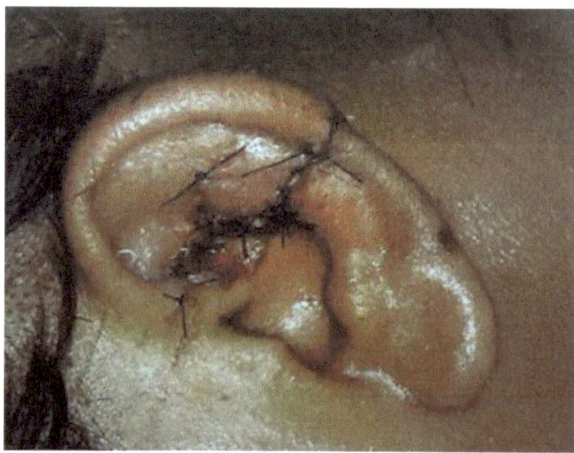

Fig. 4.6 Primary repair anteriorly

Fig. 4.7 Primary repair
posteriorly

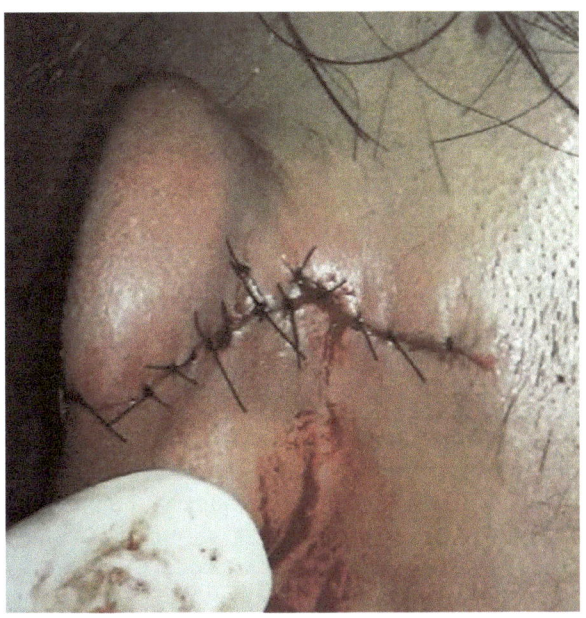

Fig. 4.8 Healed major
avulsion

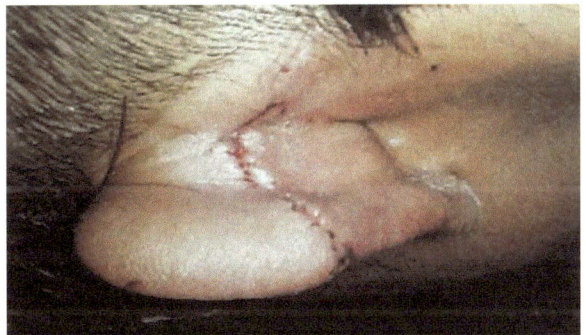

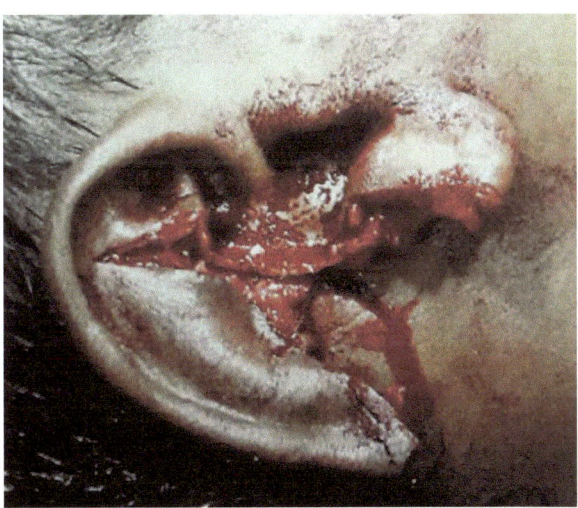

Fig. 4.9 Major avulsion
auricle

Fig. 4.10 Major avulsion
sutured

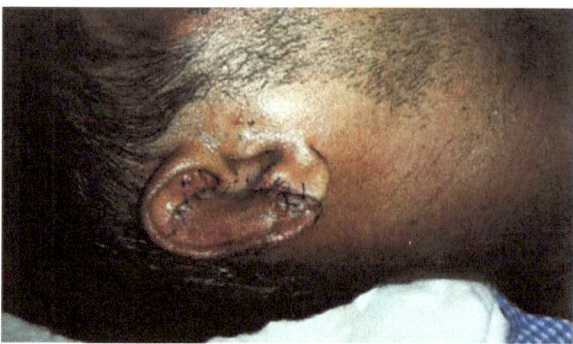

The techniques used in traumatic ear reconstruction are similar to that for
congenital ear anomalies and follow standard surgical principles [7].

4. *Complete avulsion*—when there is complete loss of the pinna, or a wound size
   larger than one and a half centimeter, bringing the skin edges together may not
   be possible. A soft tissue flap harvested from the same site, or a free flap from
   another region, may then be necessary.

Avulsion of auricle may occur with both blunt and penetrating trauma. For example,
   blunt soft tissue impact may cause enough shearing forces to tear the auricle
   apart including both the skin and the underlying cartilage. This could be seen in
   direct impact as in assault or contact sport, motor vehicle accidents with exposure of the side of head, blast trauma with shattering of soft tissue, and penetrating injury with gunshot or sharp weapons.

Loss of cartilage from the pinna results in severe scarring and distortion of anatomy.
   In certain cases, the cartilage may be present but unhealthy and devitalized and
   hence must be sacrificed. A cartilage graft from the nasal septum or rib (costal
   cartilage) may be required. These sites offer the ideal thickness of cartilage
   which may be molded into the desired shape.

For larger defects or in those patients where the general condition of the patient is
   poor or the remaining soft tissue in the area is not viable, primary repair is not
   possible. The wound may be left to heal with secondary intention, and a tertiary
   repair could be undertaken at a later stage. A prosthetic appliance may also be
   used where it is impossible to restore a normal or esthetically acceptable
   appearance.

Perichondritis of pinna may result from frostbite, thermal or chemical injury,
and radiation injury following accidental exposure or radiotherapy. It occurs due
to inflammation of the cartilage if exposed or even due to contamination of the
overlying skin resulting in infection. The affected area becomes discolored and
devitalized and is extremely tender and painful. It may lead to a spreading cellulitis of the surrounding skin and soft tissue, with the potential for hematogenous
spread of infection and sepsis in severe cases. It is thus to be detected and treated
early with antibiotics, given systemically if necessary. Failure to arrest the process
may lead to loss of tissue with cosmetic deformity or systemic complications
threatening life.

Hematoma of auricle may occur from blunt trauma as in contact sports like boxing. It may also be caused by shearing forces on the auricle as in the case of motor vehicle accidents, in which case it may be associated with abrasions over the skin and bleeding/oozing. A seroma or pseudocyst of pinna is a collection of clear or serous fluid under the skin and perichondrium of the auricular cartilage. It has no defined margins and is therefore called a pseudocyst. It is believed to be idiopathic in nature, but minor trauma such as an insect bite or scratch cannot be ruled out, and many a time a telltale sign of such trauma may be present if looked for closely.

Auricle hematomas, apart from getting infected and causing an abscess, are potentially disfiguring because the underlying cartilage undergoes aseptic necrosis and gets absorbed, thus permanently altering the appearance of the auricle. Fibrosis occurs in the spots where cartilage loss has occurred, adding to the deformity. Cosmetic reconstruction is extremely difficult and shows poor results. Recurrent hematomas lead to a deformity of the auricle known as "cauliflower ear," commonly seen in boxers. Professional sportspersons, however, are not much affected by this deformity and flaunt it as a symbol of a scintillating career in the sport.

Treatment of hematoma of auricle is similar to that of a seroma, but an open approach is recommended especially for a hematoma. Aspiration of contents followed by instillation of steroid is practiced widely but is more appropriate for seromas than traumatic hematomas. Aspiration alone might not be adequate and re-accumulation of contents is common. Incision and drainage is therefore also very common. This has the disadvantage of leaving an unsightly scar. The window technique and de-roofing of hematoma (or pseudocyst) is a more reliable technique whereby the contents can be removed properly, the cartilage inspected for areas of necrosis or devitalization and recurrence rates reduced along with a better cosmetic result [8].

Keloids are a type of hypertrophic scar where florid, uncontrolled, and lateral growth of scar occurs, leading to considerable cosmetic deformity. The word "keloid" is derived from "kelos" meaning "crab," suggesting a creeping pattern of spread, usually beyond the margins of the original wound in all directions including laterally, and therefore often visible externally. Since a keloid is a sequel to wound healing, it is best to leave it undisturbed, but treatment may be required for cosmetic and esthetic reasons. In the ear, keloids are common at the sites of ear piercing. Treatment principles have been outlined in Chap. 3.

Foreign bodies in the ear usually get impacted at the region of the isthmus of the external auditory canal, which is the narrowest part. The hairs in the outer cartilaginous part may help trap a foreign body and prevent its further progress down the canal, but some may still be found even up to the deep meatus, especially if they are animate or small, smooth, and rounded and easily able to slip inside. Inept handling of foreign bodies in the ear by inexperienced persons may cause more harm than good. Gentle syringing is generally sufficient for most foreign bodies. Insects and vegetable matter are removed more efficiently with a pair of forceps or a blunt hook. Examination and removal of a foreign body in the ear are greatly facilitated by the use of an operating microscope. The removal of the foreign body is usually carried out in the office or outpatient department without the use of anesthesia.

Smaller children may be seated in the parent or caregiver's lap, the latter making sure to cross his or her legs across the child's pelvis in order to hold it still. One arm of the adult goes around the child's shoulders and in front to keep the upper body still, while the other hand gently restrains the child's head backward and toward the opposite side. The doctor meanwhile retracts the pinna with one hand (usually the left) and removes the foreign body holding the instrument in the other hand. If the microscope is used, the child may be "mummified" by swaddling it in a thick sheet to prevent movements of the arms and legs and keeping the child still. Older children tend to struggle excessively and this method may not suffice. If the child is extremely uncooperative, it is better to remove the foreign body using a short general anesthetic agent such as ketamine or even holding down a mask if the procedure is anticipated to be easy. Impaction of the foreign body in the isthmus or deep meatus may necessitate a postaural approach under general anesthesia, especially in children. Struggling to remove the foreign body in such cases may cause it to rupture the tympanic membrane and enter the middle ear, causing predictable complications. Foreign bodies such as maggots may be removed manually after instillation of turpentine, chloroform, or liquid paraffin. Once suffocated and dead, syringing may be done to remove them en masse and debride the wound if necessary.

A variety of foreign bodies may be encountered in the head and neck region—from plastic beads and metal batteries to glue and adhesive items being introduced into the ear by unsuspecting persons. In our experience, we have come across cyanoacrylate glue (Fevistick) that was squeezed into the ear of a young girl by her illiterate father in order to relieve an earache. It ended up forming a tight mold in the ear canal and caking the facial hair outside. After managing the patient with painkillers and allowing for the glue mold to separate on its own without any sign of success, it was finally removed under general anesthesia (Fig. 4.11).

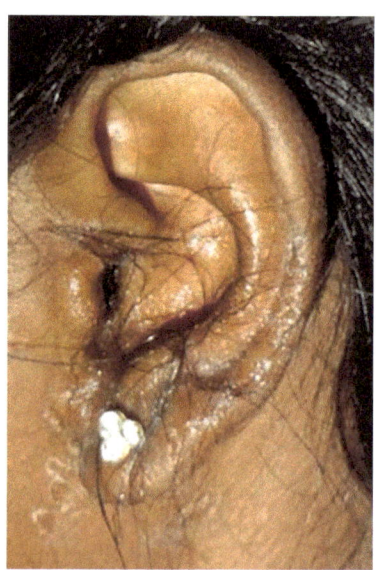

Fig. 4.11 Fevistick mold in ear canal

4.2.2   Middle Ear

Traumatic perforations of the tympanic membrane may occur as result of blunt or penetrating injury. Blunt injury occurs when the soft tissues of the lateral surface of the skull are subjected to contusion, laceration, or blast impact. This is seen in slaps or blows to the face, falls on the side of the head, and loud explosions. Penetrating trauma is seen with foreign bodies entering the ear in self-inflicted wounds by ear manipulation using fingers, ear buds, safety pins, hair clips, sticks, nails, etc. or in cases of accidents where sharp objects may find their way into the ear canal.

The perforation most commonly occurs in the anteroinferior quadrant slightly below the umbo, as this is directly in line with the forces of injury and also has the widest area of exposure where the tensile strength of the eardrum is just balanced by its fragile structure, as might be seen in any stretched membrane along its center point.

It is diagnosed by its oblong shape and irregular margins. Pain and bleeding usually occur at the onset but are not marked, while the hearing loss could be conductive or mixed depending on the impact and transmission of a pressure wave into the inner ear through the conducting apparatus. The history taking should be directed toward causation and nature of trauma and the need for establishing a medicolegal case if required. Physical examination, tuning fork tests, and pure tone audiometry are crucial. Examination under microscope (EUM) and patch test are simple means to assess the extent of damage. The edges of the perforation may be gently everted to prevent migration of squamous epithelium into the middle ear. The defect is patched with a piece of moistened Gelfoam or cigarette paper to act as a scaffold and promote rapid healing. Medication is usually not necessary in either topical or oral form. Even if no active intervention is done, medium to large traumatic perforations have the potential for complete and spontaneous repair in the absence of infection or contamination. Follow-up is important for the first 3 months to ensure that no complications have occurred and normalcy has been restored.

Ossicular discontinuity occurs due to several mechanisms. The most common is penetrating middle ear injuries and temporal bone fractures. Blast trauma and iatrogenic injuries are also seen.

The common site of discontinuity is the incudostapedial (IS) joint. Either dislocation or subluxation may occur. This results in a conductive type of hearing loss, which may be missed when other injuries of the ear are present. It usually comes to light when these are treated but the hearing loss persists. Pure tone and impedance audiometry help to establish the diagnosis. Treatment is simple and consists of exploration of the middle ear, reduction and alignment of the joint, or bridging the gap in the ossicular chain using a piece of cartilage harvested from the tragus or concha. If a lot of time has elapsed after the injury, fibrosis or ankylosis of the joint occurs and is difficult to treat. Hence a suspicion of this type of injury must always accompany trauma to the ear and be promptly treated. Established fibrosis or fixation of the joint is addressed with the use of a hearing aid.

Barotrauma can be graded from 1 to 5 on the basis of signs and symptoms, 1 being mildest and causing only discomfort without any changes in the eardrum and

5 the most severe, with perforation of the eardrum. The intermediate grades are characterized by tympanic membrane congestion, presence of fluid in the middle ear cavity, and bleeding from the capillaries in the tympanic membrane and middle ear.

Tympanic membrane congestion and capillary rupture may also occur in cases of severe hypoxia as may be seen in cases of hanging or strangulation, due to compression of the carotid artery in the neck [9]. One or both sides may be involved depending on the severity of compression. Usually as a result of such hypoxia, the victim has already been rendered unconscious. A routine ENT examination, as performed by the otolaryngologist seeing the patient, would reveal the occurrence of petechial hemorrhages on the tympanic membrane as a sign of hypoxia to the brain. Further monitoring, use of imaging such as MRI, and prognosis can be determined on the basis of this finding. This further underlines the importance of a thorough examination of a trauma victim, especially ENT, head and neck examination.

Hemotympanum is characterized by a "blue drum" due to the presence of dark blood (mainly venous) behind an intact tympanic membrane. Other causes for a blue drum are glomus tympanicum or glomus jugulare, otitis media with effusion, and cholesterol granuloma. Each of these must be differentiated on the basis of other signs and symptoms.

Middle ear barotrauma generally does not require any active treatment except for the primary or precipitating condition. An upper respiratory tract infection or allergy must be treated promptly. Active swallowing aided by chewing gum, steam inhalation, and gentle autoinflation usually suffices. Reassurance is important. Steroids may be added in individual cases where the fluid takes too long to be resorbed or the patient wishes to have a more rapid recovery.

4.2.3 Inner Ear

Barotrauma could also result in inner ear injury, causing perilymphatic fistula, labyrinthine concussion, or benign paroxysmal positional vertigo (BPPV). This occurs due to the impact of pressure disequilibrium or transmission of a pressure wave from blast trauma. The risk of perilymph fistula is greater in case of congenital weakness or anomalies of the stapes footplate or vestibular apparatus or following stapedotomy/stapedectomy. Labyrinthine concussion is a broad and nonspecific term given to inner injury due to barotraumas, resulting in a disturbance of inner ear fluids and electric potentials. Symptoms due to the above two are hearing and balance impairments, and diagnosis is more often than not delayed. Perilymph fistula must be detected and treated early to avoid permanent deafness, while labyrinthine concussion does not require any active intervention.

Labyrinthine window rupture may be explosive or implosive in nature. The implosive type is caused by a sudden increase in middle ear pressure as seen in barotraumatic otitis media, closed head injury, and blast and noise injuries. The explosive variety is due to transmission of a pressure wave through the cochlear fluids from the cerebrospinal circulation, brought about by violent sneezing, coughing, or forced Valsalva maneuver.

Intermittent and fluctuating hearing loss, with or without tinnitus and vertigo, may be seen and should raise the index of suspicion for such trauma. Examination findings and gait analysis help to differentiate between acute trauma and chronic lesions such as Meniere's disease. In the latter, the remission stages can be seen when signs and symptoms are absent. The acute stage is usually managed conservatively with or without addition of steroids. A better outcome has been reported with the intratympanic injection of autologous blood to seal the leak and may be applicable to small defects [10]. Persistence of signs and symptoms necessitates an open exploration of the middle ear contents and escape of inner ear fluids through the oval or round windows. Reverse Trendelenberg positions, use of local infiltration, or hypotensive anesthesia help to detect the leak which is then repaired. The prognosis remains poor as some amount of functional impairment has also occurred due to the leak of inner ear fluids. On the contrary, iatrogenic leak during stapedectomy is easily detected and corrected and does not result in any functional impairment in the majority of cases.

BPPV may follow traumatic insult to the inner ear and labyrinthine concussion, and the risk for this is greater with age and medical comorbidities. Whiplash is also a special kind of barotrauma but also includes mechanical and muscular trauma to the neck muscles and cervical spine and could predispose to BPPV. Knowledge of these mechanisms of injury is useful in the evaluation of BPPV, though in most cases it tends to be self-limiting.

Even without a fracture taking place, head and neck injury can occur and result in severe impairment. For example, blunt impact on the head transmits a strong pressure wave across the skull base and causes the stapes footplate to rock and thereby "shock" the inner ear fluids. This derangement takes place at the base of the cochlea and may cause a permanent hearing loss at 4 kHz. The hearing loss may also be temporary in a few cases and is then believed to have been due to a concussion injury. It may also affect the function of the peripheral vestibular apparatus and cause derangement of the fluids in the semicircular canals and otolith organs, with shearing of neurons. In either case, disturbances of balance may occur and are more difficult to recover or take a longer time to do so. The recovery is due to compensation by the healthy side and not because of return to normalcy on the affected side.

Whiplash injury of the neck may be caused by the forces of rapid acceleration and deceleration. The brainstem may also be injured by shearing and concussion in the absence of a fracture. The fibers of the 8th nerve, as well as those of the sympathetic nervous system, are affected and result in various types of central and peripheral vestibular symptoms, sometimes mimicking Meniere's disease. The latter may be a real possibility at later stages due to ischemia of the labyrinth caused by the trauma and autonomic dysfunction or shearing and tearing of the endolymphatic apparatus.

Noise-induced hearing loss refers to any kind of deafness caused by the impact of noise. It may be due to a single impact as occurs in an explosion, or due to continued exposure to high and unsafe levels of noise as occurs in industrial or occupational noise exposure, or in those staying in the vicinity of loud noise and thus being exposed. It may also occur as a result of exposure to continued low to moderate levels of noise or sound as in the use of mobile phones or recreational use of earphones to listen to music, or due to habitual and/or occupational exposure to loud music, as is seen in those working in pubs and discotheques. It may be classified as follows:

1. *Explosion*—defined as sound pressure level of 130 dB, lasting more than 3 ms, for example, grenade, industrial explosion, and airbag deployment
2. *Impulse noise injury*—defined as sound pressure level of 110–120 dB, lasting less than 3 ms, for example, gunshot, muzzle blast, and toy guns
3. *Acute acoustic trauma*—sustained but short-term exposure to sound levels of 80–100 dB, for example, recreational music at rock concerts and discotheques, personal stereos with headphones
4. *Occupational hearing loss*—seen in factories and industrial settings with continuous high ambient noise

Under normal circumstances, the acoustic or stapedial reflex helps to protect against high levels of noise by tensing the stapedial footplate against the oval window membrane, reducing movement of the ossicular chain and thus limiting the quantum of sound reaching the inner ear fluids. This reflex is active only in case of sustained exposure to high sound or noise levels and does not offer any protection against a sudden and unpredictable burst of loud sound, such as a gunshot, explosion, or the siren of an approaching train. It is also fatigable, so continued exposure to unsafe sound levels renders the stapedial reflex ineffective and predisposes to noise-induced trauma.

Loud noise is typically high-frequency sound in the range of 4–6 kHz, and thus noise injury is most commonly seen in this range. It may manifest initially with discomfort, intolerance to even normal levels of sound, pain, tinnitus, and a transient impairment of hearing. This phase is known as a temporary threshold shift because recovery to normal status is expected after about 12 h. With prolonged and repeated exposure, a permanent threshold shift appears, indicating irreversible hearing loss. The frequency of temporary threshold shift is higher in previously unexposed ears, and it is virtually impossible to predict a permanent threshold shift on the basis of how much a temporary threshold shift has occurred. High-frequency sound causes more damage than low-frequency sound, and the outer hair cells of the basal turn of the cochlea are more affected, being more directly exposed. As this is the region where the 4 kHz frequency is detected, the audiogram classically shows a notch or dip at this level. With continued noise assault over a period of time, the loss becomes more pronounced as the pillar cells, supporting cells, Reissner's membrane, and nerve fibers of the eighth cranial nerve are all affected.

Though noise-induced hearing injury is typically characterized by a high-frequency hearing loss around 4 kHz, the audiogram is not always typical. As conversational hearing levels are not affected, it is difficult to detect. Thus a screening protocol for such hearing loss exists in most industries and occupations, and workers are periodically tested with audiometry to aid early diagnosis. Sometimes, symptoms may occur in the form of tinnitus, intolerance to loud sound, or a general irritability. Depending on the level, extent, and duration of exposure, a temporary or permanent threshold shift may occur. Thus it may be reversible in the early stages and irreversible in the later stages, when it must be treated with hearing aids. Medical comorbidities and/or concomitant use of ototoxic drugs tend to complicate the situation.

Though noise trauma tends to produce a symmetric pattern of hearing loss, certain occupations and sports-related injuries as seen in rifle shooting cause an asymmetric hearing loss owing to the greater proximity of the offending source to the affected ear. Occupational hearing loss is a serious concern and is governed by strict regulations as to the permissible levels of noise and the use of protection for workers. A sound level meter is used to control noise levels in industrial settings, and worker welfares such as job rotation, surveillance, and medicolegal implications are contentious matters. Hearing is monitored regularly by pure tone audiometry, complemented with speech audiometry and brainstem evoked response audiometry (BERA) whenever required.

Occupational noise-induced hearing loss must be prevented with adequate safety measures such as provision of ear muffs to workers, control of noise and sound-proofing measures, periodic checkups, worker rotations, voluntary retirement with benefits, and compensation when indicated. Industrial ear muffs should be of a high quality so as to dampen up to 35 dB SPL (sound pressure level). Conventional or commercially available ear muffs or plugs offer less than 10 dB of sound damping and protection, so they are not useful and only serve the purpose of preventing sound transmission to the environment and reducing disturbance to others. Industrial noise exposure is subject to regulation and is usually followed uniformly in all countries. In short, the cutoff hazard point is 90 dB, and a full day's work or shift duty for this level of ambient noise should not exceed 8 h. The time is exponentially reduced thereafter for every 5 dB increase in the sound level. Thus, only 4 h of exposure are permissible for 95 dB, 2 h for 100 dB, 1 h for 105 dB, half an hour for 110 dB, and 15 min for 115 dB.

If hearing loss has occurred, disability may be calculated by the formula given below according to the AMA (American Medical Association) method formulated in the year 1979. The normal threshold is taken to be 25 dB.

Right (or better) ear impairment = 1.5 (hearing threshold in decibels − 25) = figure in percentage

Left (or worse) ear impairment = 1.5 (hearing threshold in decibels − 25) = figure in percentage

Hearing handicap (HH) or binaural impairment (BI) = 5/6 (percentage for better ear) + 1/6 (percentage for worse ear)

For example, if the hearing threshold for the worse ear is 40 dB and that for the better ear 30, then the hearing handicap would be calculated as follows:

$1.5(30 − 25) (5/6) + 1.5(40 − 25) (1/6) = 10\%$ hearing disability

4.2.4 Facial Nerve

Electrodiagnostic tests for facial paralysis have a great prognostic value if the correct parameters are used. These are the velocity of onset of complete paralysis (time course), the end point of denervation (maximal value) and the early return of voluntary function or movements (early deblocking). Serial tests must be done in order to decide the exact point at which surgical intervention might be necessary. This principle applies equally to major trauma to the temporal bone as well as in iatrogenic injuries to the nerve [11].

The nerve excitability test (NET) uses a threshold stimulus to measure nerve function at the facial nerve root as it emerges at the stylomastoid foramen. A difference of 3.5 milliamperes (mA) between the two sides is considered significant, although an absolute increase of 150% over the normal is also considered significant by some [12].

The maximal stimulation test (MST) as the name suggests stimulates the individual branches of the nerve over the facial musculature using a supramaximal stimulus of up to a maximum of 1 mA to evoke maximal response, and the difference in response in the two sides is calculated in increments of 25%, up to 100% of the normal side. The test is painful and uncomfortable for some patients, so a minimum time period of stimulation of 400 ms instead of 1 millisecond (ms) is considered optimal [13].

The electroneurography (ENoG) test uses maximal stimulation at the nerve root and measures the compound muscle action potentials (CMAP) at the end organ. It may thus be considered an evoked electromyography (EEMG). A difference of 3% between the two sides is normal, and more than a difference of 30% in the response against the normal side is considered sufficient for surgical intervention in order to ensure a fair outcome. The speed at which the worsening of the affected side occurs (up to 5% preservation of function—or 95% degeneration—over 2 weeks bodes for a poor outcome or just about 50% chances of recovery of function) [14].

Electromyography (EMG) measures the function of the motor end plates of the facial musculature. Fibrillation potentials appear after about 2 weeks following denervation, but gradually polyphasic action potentials are seen to emerge at 4–6 weeks, signifying return of function by fibers of the regenerating neurons. In traumatic facial palsy presenting late, this test is used to determine if dynamic reinnervation procedures such as nerve grafts or nerve muscle transfers wound be useful.

Electrodiagnostic tests are useful after about 3 weeks of injury when there is no clinical improvement visible and the viability of the nerve is in question. Prior to this period, it is only justified if the paralysis is of immediate onset and complete in nature, and there is evidence of total transection of the nerve on imaging. The test of choice is evoked electromyography (EEMG), also known as electroneurography (ENoG), which is expected to show that more than 90% of the nerve fibers have been damaged and Wallerian degeneration has set in. In established cases of nerve paralysis, an electromyography (EMG) may also be done to look for polyphasic action potentials which signify viable motor end plates and good muscle function, or fibrillation potentials which indicate that the motor end plates are not conducting impulses and the enervated muscles have undergone atrophy.

Wallerian degeneration takes time to occur even in a fully transected nerve, so the nerve continues to transmit impulses and may provide a false-positive result on facial nerve electromyography [15].

The main limitation of electrical tests is that they are not a 100% reliable in all cases as loss of function in the nerve may be of the mixed variety, with some having neuropraxia and some being structurally disrupted.

Other less commonly used tests are antidromic test, stapedial reflex evoked potential, facial nerve stimulation and nerve monitoring, nerve muscle biopsy, and the topodiagnostic tests, namely, the Schirmer's test, salivary flow test, taste sensation measurements, and estimation of salivary pH.

Imaging plays a crucial role in facial nerve paralysis due to any cause and particularly in trauma. The portion of nerve involved, the presence of edema or hematoma, or impinging bone fragments are best seen on CT scanning, especially high-resolution CT scanning (HRCT) using 0.8–1 mm fine cuts in both axial and coronal views. The axial view is especially useful for the geniculate ganglion and horizontal portion of the facial nerve, while the coronal view is useful for the vertical portion of the nerve and as well as for detecting fractures of the skull base or tegmen plate (Figs. 4.12, 4.13, 4.14, 4.15, 4.16).

MRI is not considered useful as bony injuries are not picked up well with this modality and is only indicated if any other lesion such as brain damage is to be determined. The area of the geniculate ganglion of the facial nerve (GGF) is most vulnerable to trauma as it lies just beyond the labyrinthine segment and it is this portion that must be especially looked for on imaging.

The degree and nature of treatment for facial nerve injury must be customized to the specific needs of the individual patient [16]. Subtle factors would play crucial roles in the decision-making and one size does not fit all.

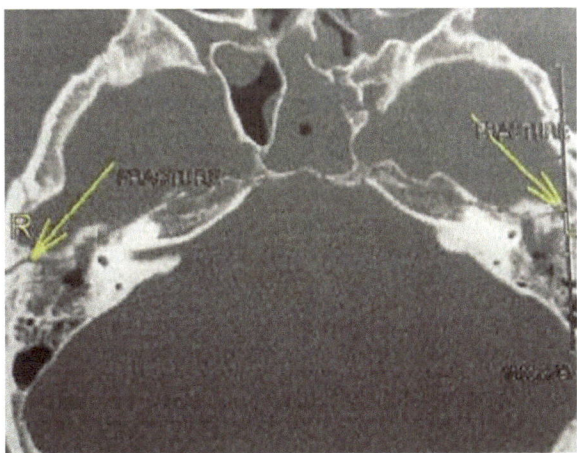

Fig. 4.12 Transverse fracture

Fig. 4.13 OCV type of
fracture

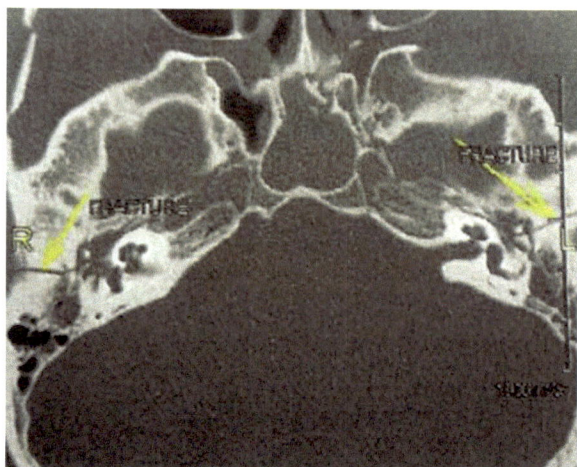

Fig. 4.14 Facial nerve;
geniculate ganglion

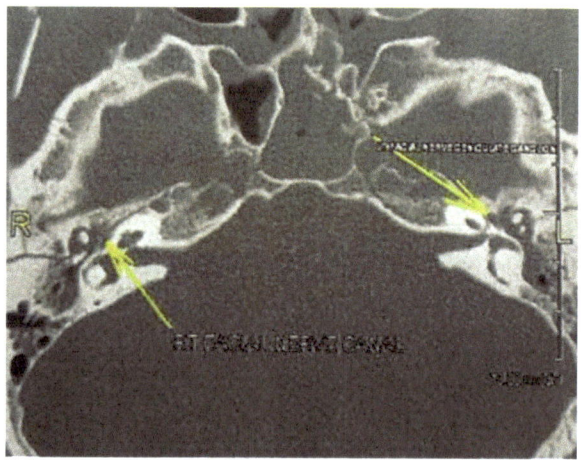

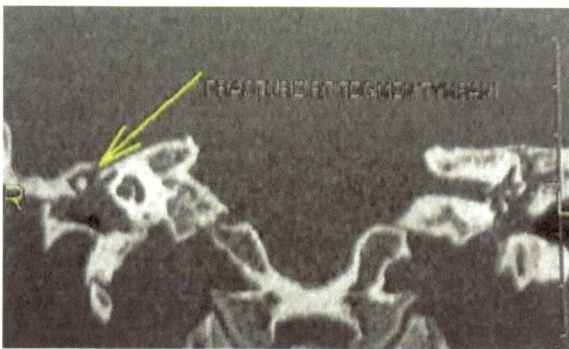

Fig. 4.15 Coronal view;
tegmen fracture

Fig. 4.16 Multiple
tegmen fractures

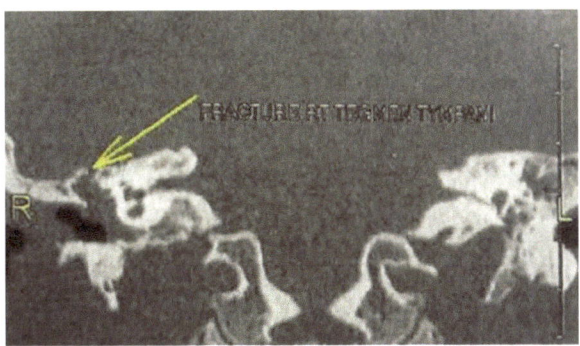

If delayed facial palsy or paresis has occurred, it may be due to concussion following the initial impact, or ischemia leading to nerve sheath edema and subsequent compression, or even a granuloma or granulations that have formed as a result of continued edema and inflammation and/or infection. Temporal bone fractures in which immediate or early facial nerve paralysis occurs require a different approach toward management. Such injuries would be evident on imaging and warrant early surgical intervention in the form of facial nerve decompression and/or direct repair as soon as the patient has been stabilized.

A delayed presentation, on the other hand, usually responds to a conservative approach with medical management, eye care, and active and passive physiotherapy in the form of galvanic stimulation, facial exercises, and massage. The treatment of facial nerve paralysis in the early stages or for less severe grades of injury may also be conservative and involve medical management in the form of corticosteroids principally and antivirals and antibacterials as supplementary medications. If no recovery occurs over at least 3 weeks, then electrophysiological tests are needed to demonstrate if Wallerian degeneration is taking place. In such an event, open surgical exploration may be justified, but the patient is to be given a guarded prognosis.

Eye care is given by performing a temporary closure of the eye by doing a tarsorrhaphy which may be medial, lateral, or central. In established cases, a lid loading with gold weight or a lid tightening procedure (blepharoplasty) as part of a face lift may be carried out. Other ways in which lid closure may be augmented are the use of spacer grafts, or doing a lateral tarsal strip procedure which shortens the horizontal aperture of the eye, or a lateral transorbital canthopexy procedure which does not result in shortening of the horizontal aperture.

Even though steroids lower the threshold for seizure occurrence in cases of head injury, associated complete facial palsy does benefit immensely from the use of steroids and must be considered whenever possible [17].

Primary repair may be carried out by doing an end-to-end anastomosis if the length of the gap is 2 cm or less or an interposition or transposition procedure if longer segments are involved or missing. Primary repair of the facial nerve may be carried out surgically by nerve grafting. The sural nerve may be used as a sensory nerve graft as it provides the maximum length of up to 35 cm, with minimal morbidity to the donor site [18]. The sural nerve is the nerve of choice for grafting as it provides a length of up to 35 cm. The great auricular nerve and the antecubital or cutaneous communicating nerves are other sources of graft material.

Options to grafting include nerve transfer or nerve muscle transfer, both of which provide speedier results than those provided by nerve grafting. The opposite facial, masseteric, hypoglossal, and spinal accessory nerves may be used for nerve transfer. The muscles that may be used for a nerve muscle transfer include the temporalis muscle along with its tendon, which may be harvested locally, or the pectoralis minor, latissimus dorsi, rectus abdominis or gracilis, which are obtained as free muscle transfers. When facial nerve injury is complete and irreversible, a minimally invasive temporalis muscle tendon transfer can be performed in an orthodromic fashion, with a 2 cm incision in the nasolabial fold [19]. Alternatively, a fully intraoral approach may be used. Adequate tension on the tendon is desirable in order to optimize outcomes. An allograft nerve of up to 7 cm is also commercially available and may be used in cases where autograft material is not available. All these methods are aimed toward providing dynamic reanimation of the facial musculature.

Gold weights or implants are a convenient method of static reanimation of the affected face following facial nerve damage due to injury or other causes. This is mainly done with the purpose of maintaining facial symmetry when smiling and also at rest and may be combined with dynamic reanimation procedures. Gold weights are available or can be customized in weights ranging from 0.6 to 2.8 g to suit different patients or situations, but commonly the weight of the implant ranges from 0.6 to 1.8 g depending on the age, sex, and build of the patient. The thickness is approximately 0.6 mm, while the diameter is 12 mm. A circular or elliptical shape is cosmetically more acceptable.

It is inserted in the preseptal or pretarsal space using a linear incision under local anesthesia. The optimal location of the implant is the junction of the medial and central part of the eyeball because here the eye closure brought about by the implant is perfectly counterbalanced by the opening action of the levator palpebrae muscle. The weight of the implant necessary may be determined preoperatively by titrating a silastic mold or models of various sizes and weights by temporarily fixing them on the upper eyelid using micropore strips. The eye closure seen on the affected side with the weight in place must be at least 1 mm more compared to the normal or unaffected eye, with the patient facing and looking straight ahead. The implant is ideally centered in the middle of the upper eyelid for best results. Siting it deeper in the eyelid may hide the contours of the implant and offer a better appearance, but this may be suboptimal for eye closure. Bringing it closer to the lid margin will improve closure but make the implant more obvious and therefore less acceptable to the patient.

Miscellaneous procedures to improve facial function and esthetic appearance may be required in certain patients. These include a brow lift, midface or full-face lifts, and augmentation with autologous fat. Synkinesis is a serious problem in higher grades of nerve paralysis, and this is tackled using techniques such as directed chemo-denervation or division of the platysma in the neck (platysmectomy). Physiotherapy plays a crucial role in long-term rehabilitation and includes patient education, relaxation exercises, biofeedback, mechanical/ manual stimulation (massage), stress integration, facial strengthening, face tapping, specific action, eyelid-specific exercises, and electrical stimulation. Supplementation with vitamins B12 and B1 is also useful.

4.3 Best Practice Recommendations

- *Prevention* is the key to the avoidance of barotrauma. Proper training of pilots and deep sea divers, gradual descent and ascent, prompt treatment of nasal pathology, good nasal hygiene, and use of decongestants in vulnerable individuals prior to flight or dive are adequate measures.
- *Labyrinthine concussion or rupture* may be initially missed in the light of more grave injuries and prolonged bed rest, immobilization and hospitalization mean that much of the functional impairment caused by the labyrinthine injury is resolved by the process of compensation by the time the patient is up and about. If imbalance and/or hearing loss persist, surgical exploration for a perilymph leak may be undertaken.
- *Workers' rights and information* about industrial noise exposure are widely available on the government and labor union websites in virtually all countries. Disability is calculated using mathematical formulae in order to determine corrective action, rehabilitation, and compensation.
- *Facial nerve and labyrinthine injuries* are common in OCV fractures. Immediate and complete facial paralysis warrants an early surgical intervention especially if imaging studies reveal hematoma, bony spicules, or transection of the nerve. Cases of delayed facial weakness usually manifest as a paresis and not complete paralysis and may be managed conservatively with steroids in oral or parenteral form, eye care, and facial physiotherapy—both active and passive. Electrophysiological studies and advanced imaging studies like a high-resolution CT scan (HRCT) are useful for monitoring the progress of the facial nerve injury, and surgical decompression may be justified if signs of degeneration are evident. Both static and dynamic reanimation procedures may be used alone or in combination to restore normalcy to the face.
- *Trauma to the ear* may include the outer ear (hematoma of auricle, seroma, cauliflower ear, avulsion of auricle, frostbite with perichondritis, and keloids), middle ear (traumatic perforation, ossicular discontinuity, barotraumas, perilymph fistula, BPPV, labyrinthine concussion), inner ear (blast trauma, noise-induced hearing loss, temporal bone fractures), and surgical trauma. While some of these require very simple treatment, others would necessarily involve multidisciplinary management. Understanding of the nature of these injuries is crucial to optimizing outcomes.

Conclusion

Ear trauma is best understood and optimally managed by keeping in mind its divisions into the outer, middle, and inner ears.

References

1. Weerda H. Chirurgie der Ohrmuschel Verletzungen, Defekte und Anomalien. Stuttgart: Thieme; 2004. p. 105–226.
2. Ihrai T, Balaquer T, Monteil MC, Chignon-Sicard B, Medard de Chardon V, Riah Y, Lebreton E. Surgical management of traumatic ear amputations: literature review. Ann Chir Plast Esthet. 2009;54(2):146–51.
3. Wong W, Wilson P, Savundra J. Total ear replantation using the distal radial artery perforator. J Plast Reconstr Aesthet Surg. 2011;64(5):677–9.
4. Saad Ibrahim SM, Zidan A, Madani S. Totally avulsed ear: new technique of immediate ear reconstruction. J Plast Reconstr Anesthet Surg. 2008;61(Suppl 1):S29–36.
5. Horta R, Costa-Ferreira A, Costa J, Silva P, Amarante JM, Silva A, Filipe R. Ear replantation after human bite avulsion injury. J Craniofac Surg. 2011;22(4):1457–9.
6. Norman ZI, Cracchiolo JR, Allen SH, Soliman AMS. Auricular reconstruction after human bite amputation using the Baudet technique. Ann Otol Rhinol Laryngol. 2014;124(1):45–8.
7. Siegert R, Magritz R. Reconstruction of the auricle. GMS Curr Top Otorhinolaryngol Head Neck Surg. 2007;6:Doc 02. Epub 2008 Mar 14.
8. Kanotra SP, Lateef M. Preudocyst of pinna: a recurrence-free approach. Am J Otolaryngol. 2009;30(2):73–9.
9. Rasmussen ER, Larsen PL, Andersen K, Larsen M, Qvortrup K, Hougen HP. Petechial hemorrhages of the tympanic membrane in attempted suicide by hanging: a case report. J Forensic Legal Med. 2013;20(2):119–21.
10. Foster PK. Autologous intratympanic blood patch for presumed perilymphatic fistulas. J Laryngol Otol. 2016;130:1158–61.
11. Fisch U. Prognostic value of electrical tests in acute facial paralysis. Am J Otol. 1984;5(6):494–8.
12. Mechelse K, Huizing EH, Van Bolhuis AH, Goor G, Hammelburg E, Staal A, Verjaal A. Bell's palsy: prognostic criteria and evaluation of surgical decompression. Lancet. 1971;298(7715):57–60.
13. Molina P, Bertrand RA, Hardy J. The trigemino-facial reflexes. In: Fisch U, editor. Facial nerve surgery. Amstelveen: Kugler Medical Publications; 1977. p. 107–23.
14. Esslen E. The acute facial palsies. Berlin: Springer-Verlag; 1977. p. 7–8.
15. Sittel C, Stennert E. Prognostic value of electromyography in acute peripheral facial nerve palsy. Otol Neurotol. 2001;22:100–4.
16. Greywoode JD, Ho HH, Artz GJ. Management of traumatic facial nerve injuries. Facial Plast Surg. 2010;26:511–8.
17. Hadlock T. Facial paralysis: research and future directions. Facial Plast Surg. 2008;24:260–7.
18. Humphrey CD, Kriet JD. Nerve repair and cable grafting for facial paralysis. Facial Plast Surg. 2008;24:170–6.
19. Boahene KD, Farrag TY, Ishii L, Byrne PJ. Minimally invasive temporalis tendon transposition. Arch Facial Plast Surg. 2011;13:8–13.

Trauma to the Nose and Face

5

Learning Objectives
- To learn the pathophysiology of trauma to the nose and facial skeleton
- To understand the clinical implications of management of trauma to the nose and face
- To remember the best practice recommendations in nasal and facial trauma

5.1 Pathophysiology

5.1.1 Embryology, Anatomy, and Biomechanics

The nose starts to develop from the nasal placodes in the fourth week of gestation and reaches adult structure and function by birth, though it continues to grow up to adulthood with development of both the skeletal and soft tissue components. Interference with the skeletal elements such as the bone and cartilage may hamper its growth with respect to the rest of the facial skeleton; thus both injuries to the nose and surgical procedures on the nose before 18 years of age have serious impact upon it. It is also the most projected and prominent part of the face and is thus especially vulnerable to trauma. It also has a rich vascular supply, and injury of any kind is likely to result bleeding of variable severities depending on the site and force involved. The soft tissues of the nose and the mucosa both tend to bleed easily in trauma especially if there are comorbidities such as bleeding abnormalities, high blood pressure, and atherosclerosis or if the patient is taking anticoagulant medications.

In children the development of the facial skeleton is unique and different from that in adults. One of the most important aspects is the face-to-cranium ratio, which is 1:8 at birth and reaches 1:2 in adulthood. Thus most of the growth of the face is in the vertical direction and brought about by the development of the alveoli and the

© Springer Nature Singapore Pte Ltd. 2018
J. Das, *Trauma in Otolaryngology*, https://doi.org/10.1007/978-981-10-6361-9_5

eruption of teeth. Also, lack of pneumatization of the mandible in a child renders it stiffer and more elastic and thus better able to withstand injury. The elasticity is provided by the preponderance of cancellous over cortical bone and a greater amount of subcutaneous fat making the skin and soft tissue more thick and supple. The teeth appear around 6 months of age, and the primary or deciduous dentition is achieved by 2 years of age. Between 6 and 12 years, the permanent dentition is completed, while the wisdom teeth or last molars appear by 18 years of age but may be unerupted, partially erupted, or impacted in some people.

5.1.2   Nasal Septum

The nose is subjected to trauma right at the time of inception of the human birth process as the baby passes through the stages of labor. As molding takes place in the second stage of labor, the nasal septum is also subjected to stresses and strains. Being soft and elastic in nature, the nasal septal cartilage is held under tension by the overlying mucoperichondrial flaps on either side of it, but any impact or injury on these surfaces can affect the shape of the septum. This is known as the Fry principle. Trauma caused by the compressive forces of molding results in microfractures of the septal cartilage and changes such as telescoping, duplication, scarring, and spur formation, thus leading to septal deviations. This is called Gray's birth molding theory.

As the child grows into adolescence and then adulthood, these changes become more pronounced. Additional changes such as turbinate hypertrophy may occur, further compounding the nasal airway narrowing and obstruction present due to the deviated nasal septum. So even though this condition is developmental in nature, the root cause is trauma sustained during birth.

As the facial skeleton is constantly in a state of flux and molding up to the age of 18, minimal intervention is advised when trauma occurs prior to this age. Surgical treatment, if aggressive, may be counterproductive. It is necessary to ensure that no significant deformity occurs and nasal patency and function are maintained. However, gross external deformity may be corrected as soon as possible, and fine-tuning of traumatic deformities is best undertaken when full growth has occurred and has stabilized. In these cases, a septorhinoplasty and other forms of facial reconstructive and cosmetic correction can be done.

Digital trauma to the nose is more common than believed. Children of all ages are natural explorers and the nasal cavities are their favorite sites! Insertion of foreign bodies apart, nose picking is particularly common and is exacerbated as much by dry, dusty conditions as by attacks of rhinitis and runny nose. Nose picking in children traumatizes the retro-columellar vein which is not only delicate but also very prominent and vascular in young children. The bleeding is brisk but usually stops spontaneously unless local infection in the form of rhinitis, or a bleeding disorder, is present. Adults are also often given to nose picking or worse, nose digging, and this is more common where there is an underlying sensation of irritation caused by dryness and crusting, as is likely to happen in cases of a deviated nasal septum with spur.

Nose picking, and the use of snuff and recreational drugs taken by inhalation, for example cocaine, can cause traumatic perforations of the nasal septum, both as a direct effect and also because of ischemic necrosis. Tattoos and piercings on the face are other lesser discussed forms of trauma. Both of these are used for cosmetic and recreational purposes, but if not done with aseptic precautions, they may get infected leaving a scar and result in deformity due to keloid formation or perichondritis.

5.1.3 Nasal Bones

The nasal bones may be fractured by a lateral force causing a vertical type I fracture also known as a Chevallet fracture or by a frontal force causing a C-shaped type II fracture known as a Jarjavay fracture. Both these types of injury not only involve the nasal bones but also the nasal septum which is tethered to the nasal bones on either side. A Chevallet fracture causes a linear fracture of the septum from the dorsum to the floor due to the lateral impact. A Jarjavay fracture is caused by a frontal impact on the nose, causing the nasal septum to buckle backward and give way in a breach that assumes a curvilinear shape from the dorsal nasal spine through the perpendicular plate of the ethmoid and septal cartilage to the floor of the nose and then anteriorly to end at the maxillary crest and the inferior (anterior) nasal spine.

Both may result in the formation of a septal hematoma, but the second type causes a greater displacement of the fracture fragments and collapse or deformity of the nasal dorsum.

5.1.4 Facial Skeleton

The face is composed of many different bones aligned with each other, some strong, some delicate, and all encompassing a myriad of structures including blood vessels and nerves. The various bones include the paired maxillae; the zygomatic, lacrimal, nasal, ethmoid, inferior turbinate and palatine bones; the frontal bone, vomer, and sphenoid in the center with its two pterygoid plates; and the zygomatic processes of the temporal bones on either side. It is easy to appreciate the complexity of such anatomy and its implications for the trauma surgeon as far as restoration to the normal is concerned.

Trauma to the region of the oral cavity may cause internal injuries involving the mucosal surfaces, and external injury may not be obvious. Mucosal injury is greater as there is contiguity of the bone and soft tissue in many areas, for example, at the junction of the gum margins and palate. As the submucosa is extremely vascular, hematomas may form with even minor degrees of trauma, resulting in pain and difficulty in opening the mouth, chewing, and swallowing. A meticulous examination of the mucosal surfaces is thus very important even in the absence of bleeding or external deformity. The alveolar margins should also be carefully examined for missing or loose teeth, impaction of teeth, bone or foreign particles, and deep mucosal injuries connecting the oral cavity to the nasal and sinus cavities. The presence of subcutaneous emphysema may be due to communication with the airway or external environment and is an important clinical indicator of impending airway obstruction and the onset of infection of the fascial spaces or soft tissue cellulitis.

The strength of the facial skeleton is derived from the vertical and horizontal buttresses which maintain height and projection, respectively. The vertical buttress is formed by the frontal bone principally along with the maxillae and zygomatic bones, while the horizontal buttresses are formed by the upper and lower alveoli and the supraorbital ridges of the orbit.

The face can be divided into three zones:

1. *The upper one third* includes the frontal sinuses and frontal bone up to the level of the eyebrows.

   In this region, clinical examination should rule out bony depressions and step deformities over the forehead and lacerations of the skin and soft tissue. The frontal bone is strong and able to withstand the considerable forces inflicted by trauma. Usually it is the outer table of the frontal sinuses that is vulnerable to fracture, and the likelihood of this is increased if the frontal sinuses are hypoplastic and not fully developed or pneumatized. Fracture of both tables of the frontal sinus results in penetration into the intracranial cavity and may lead to herniation of the brain and cerebrospinal fluid (CSF) leak.

2. *The middle third* composed of the nose, eyes, naso-orbito-ethmoid (NOE) complex, the two maxillae and zygomatic bones, and the palate.

   On clinical examination, facial asymmetry is evident if proptosis (increase in the vertical dimension) or enophthalmos (decrease in the anteroposterior dimension) is present. Though this is usually seen on direct examination, an indirect evidence of the same is provided if the upper lid crease is increased (deepened) or there is an increase in the length of the upper lid. The presence of enophthalmos can also be detected by applanation tonometry, which would reveal a pressure difference of more than 4 mm Hg. The forced duction test is also a useful clinical method to determine mobility of the globe and entrapment of intraocular muscle in an orbital blowout fracture. To do this, the conjunctiva must first be anesthetized using a topical agent, and then the globe can be moved in all directions and restriction of movement observed in the direction of involved muscle. The medial canthus of the eye can be grasped, at the point of its attachment on the sclera, between forceps to judge firmness or loss of elasticity, which would suggest avulsion of the medial canthus from its attachment. Though it is rare for the medial canthus to be completely avulsed or detached, the more common occurrence is that it exerts traction on its bony attachment, which in turn is gradually displaced from its normal position, thus changing the final resting position of the globe. A negative forced duction test also helps to differentiate entrapment of the medial rectus muscle from ophthalmoplegia. In the latter, the globe can be passively moved while this is not possible in case of muscle entrapment.

3. *The lower third* that is mainly composed of the mandible is visualized best using a combination of CT scan imaging and an orthopantomogram (OPG), as both of

these provide useful information about different sites of the mandible being involved by the trauma.

The facial skeleton may be subject to external physical forces from virtually all aspects—frontal (anteroposterior), lateral, frontolateral, cephalocaudal, and torsional. The force required to cause fractures in the facial skeleton varies from 300 to 900 kg per square centimeter. Injuries may thus impact one or many bones along with their respective soft tissue structures, and the quantum of injury may vary considerably. Common patterns of injury have been identified in the following sections. The clinical presentation of each is given alongside.

Facial fractures could also be classified as those involving the median structures and those involving the paramedian or lateral structures. Thus, frontal sinus, nasal, oral, and oropharyngeal trauma would be distinctly different from fractures of the maxillae, mandible, or orbit. This helps to identify the specialties dealing with each of these types of trauma. While the median sites would be in the purview of the ENT specialist, the others would be dealt with by the plastic and reconstructive surgeon, maxillofacial surgeon, or ophthalmologist. But more often than not, a multispecialty approach is required, and each site may be addressed by one or more persons at the same or subsequent sittings. Nevertheless, most of the discussion shall reiterate these classical patterns of facial trauma in order to streamline it. It must be borne in mind at all times that clinical assessment of each individual case must override any kind of textbook description given anywhere.

5.1.5 The Le Fort Types of Injuries

The Le Fort types of injuries pertain to the midface and are a simplistic way of classifying trauma to this region. Needless to say, any one of these is rarely found in its typical description but rather as a mixed type. What is important is to be able to clinically assess the structures involved, the mode of investigation required to establish a diagnosis, and the treatment thereof.

The Le Fort type 1 fracture is known as the Guerin fracture and is the least common. A very severe degree of injury, known as the type 4 fracture, is also very uncommon and is said to occur in the coronal plane of the base of the skull. It is more likely to be a combination of the other types of Le Fort fractures. The type 2 is the most common followed by the type 3 in case of severe trauma. The latter may even be fatal as it involves skull base fractures and a severe form of traumatic brain injury in the majority of cases. Airway obstruction is also a major risk in type 3 and 4 fractures, and in suspected cases, the upper jaw may be manually pulled forward as a first-aid measure to maintain respiration.

Le Fort 1:

In this type, the impact is usually low velocity and anteroposterior in direction, causing the fracture line to pass along the floor of the nasal cavity and the margins of the upper alveolus and extending backward to the base of the vomer and the perpendicular plates of the palatine bones. Thus it separates the lower third of the nasal septum and the maxillary teeth in the center and on both sides the medial and lateral walls of the maxillary sinuses from the pterygoid plates and palatine bones posteriorly. Personal assault, falls, sports injuries, and minor vehicular accidents are common causes.

Epistaxis, pain on opening the mouth, malocclusion, loose or broken teeth, and external deformity are the usual symptoms. Bruising or contusion of the skin and soft tissues, mucosal hematomas in the oral cavity, crepitations over the bony prominences, and mobility of some segments of the maxillary alveolus along with loose or lost teeth are the usual signs. An anterior overbite may be evident. Two fingers (index and middle) may be inserted into the oral cavity to palpate the posterior margin of the palate which would be found to have a breach and allow a degree of mobility but not be completely dislocated.

Le Fort 2:

In this type, the degree of impact is greater and the direction may be frontal, frontolateral, lateral, or torsional. The fracture line passes obliquely across the medial aspect of the maxillae and the nasal processes of the frontal bone and backward across the alveoli, vomer, palate, and pterygoid processes. Thus it separates the nasal, lacrimal, and ethmoid bones in the center and the maxillary complexes at the zygoma on both sides, from the pterygoid plates and the base of the skull posteriorly. Assault with a heavy or blunt weapon, fall from a height, occupational injuries and low-velocity vehicular accidents are the usual causes.

All the symptoms of the first type, as well as significant external deformity and soft tissue injury, along with gagging, trismus, blurring of vision and double vision, and loss of sensation over the face, may be present. Raccoon eyes, subconjunctival hemorrhage, diplopia, restricted movement of the globe(s), mobile maxillae or nasal bones, anterior open bite, and facial anesthesia are the usual signs. Using the two fingers in the mouth again, considerable movement of the bones may be confirmed even though they are still attached to the facial skeleton.

Le Fort 3:

In this type, the force of injury is massive, as might be seen in complex, high-velocity trauma such as motor vehicle accidents or industrial injuries, which are the usual causes. The fracture line passes through the nasal, ethmoid, and orbital bones and the zygomaticomaxillary complex into the pterygopalatine and sphenopalatine fossae. Thus it separates the facial skeleton from the base of the skull and is known as craniofacial disjunction.

All the symptoms of the first two types, as also cerebrospinal fluid (CSF) rhinorrhea and gross deformity, may be present. The physical examination would reveal signs common to the first two types and separation of the midface from the skull— or craniofacial disjunction due to a rift at the zygomaticofrontal suture line—confirmed by inserting two fingers into the throat.

Swelling, soft tissue lacerations, loss of sensation or abnormal sensation, loss or impaction of teeth, and epistaxis with or without cerebrospinal fluid (CSF) leak are thus symptoms common to both Le Fort 2 and 3 types of fractures and also involvement of other bones with various other patterns of injury. Mucosal tears or lacerations, and abnormal mobility or malocclusion, are also clinical signs that are common to both.

5.1.6 Fronto-ethmoid Complex

The frontal bone, being strong and stout in nature, does not fracture easily. The outer table may break with direct impact from the anterior direction, and the fragment may be depressed, thus causing a deformity, in which case it needs to be corrected. Fracture of the thinner inner table may not be evident unless there is a CSF leak. A CT scan may be ordered if serious injury to the frontal sinus is suspected.

A fronto-ethmoid fracture may cause pseudohypertelorism or telecanthus if the medial canthal ligaments are avulsed and true hypertelorism if there is an accompanying fracture of the ethmoid complex. Open reduction and internal fixation (ORIF) techniques are required in such cases employing various methods such as wires, screws, and plates. Anterior nasal packing alone may suffice in a handful of instances where no significant displacement, comminuting fragments, or deformity has occurred.

Fractures of the naso-orbito-ethmoid (NOE) complex are divided into the following:

1. *Grade 1*—fracture without injury to the medial canthal ligament, with minimal or no displacement
2. *Grade 2*—as above but the displaced fragment can be reduced, that is, fracture with injury to the medial canthal ligament but without its complete avulsion
3. *Grade 3*—as above but the displaced fragment cannot be reduced, that is, fracture with injury to the medial canthal ligament with complete avulsion

The medial canthus, also known as the medial canthal tendon or medial canthal ligament, is attached in front to the frontal process of the maxilla just in front of the lacrimal groove and behind to the lacrimal bone. On either side, it is also attached to the tarsus muscle of the upper and lower eyelids and is roughly 2 mm wide and 4 mm long.

Hypertelorism refers to an increase in the interpupillary distance over the normal distance of 60 mm and involves an absolute increase in the bony dimensions between the two orbits. This may be seen in developmental disorders such as ethmoid polyposis or fibrous dysplasia, especially in the growing facial skeleton of children and young adolescents. *Telecanthus* is an apparent increase to about 45 mm in the distance between the two globes over the normal distance of 30 mm and is caused by extensive soft tissue injury and edema over the root of the nose. Both, however, lead to facial asymmetry and disfigurement.

Such injuries may also cause disruption of the orbital exoskeleton and lead to entrapment of the muscle, namely the inferior rectus more commonly or inferior oblique less commonly, and the medial rectus, causing extraocular movements to be restricted in the direction of action of the involved muscle. Blowout fractures also cause loss of orbital fat, making the orbital contents prolapse posteriorly, inferiorly, and medially, leading to sinking of the eyeball into the orbit, also known as enophthalmos or hypoglobus.

5.1.7 Zygomaticomaxillary Complex

Different types of classification of zygomatic fractures are in use, and one of the most useful is that which recognizes four types according to the site and bone(s) involved, thus giving direction to the clinical management of these fractures [1].

Zygomatic fractures follow such lines of disruption because of the inherent lines of weakness of the facial skeleton [2].

Fractures of the zygomaticomaxillary complex (ZMC) may thus be divided into zygomaticofrontal (superiorly), zygomaticomaxillary (anteromedial/inferior), zygomaticotemporal (posterolateral), and zygomaticosphenoid (posteromedial). Tripod or tetrapod fractures may be seen with involvement of three or four fragments and also comminuted fractures with multiple fragments.

Fractures of the zygoma, or malar complex, may be encountered with frontal or laterally directed impact and are relatively more common as the cheek forms the most prominent part of the face and thus is most vulnerable to the external environment. Soft tissue contusion may mask such fractures, so a high index of suspicion must be maintained. There may a step deformity of the infraorbital rim, and imaging studies would help confirm this. The infraorbital nerve may also be involved, causing anesthesia of the cheek.

5.1.8 Mandible

Fractures may also involve only the upper and lower jaws when the force is extremely lateral, causing maxillary-mandibular fractures, and also the hard palate in isolation, as seen in Le Fort 1, or palatal fractures caused by intraoral injury, such as that due to the accidental and forceful impaction of a foreign body, for example a pencil held in the mouth.

Fractures of the mandible or jawbone are commonly associated with fractures of the facial skeleton and may occur in about 50% of such injuries. The rounded shape of the mandible creates several points of weakness, the weakest being the condyle of the mandible. Thus condylar fractures are the most common, followed by fractures of the angle and the symphysis menti.

The fracture may involve the condyle, ramus, angle, symphysis or body of the mandible, or the tooth roots (dentoalveolar). Care must be exercised to avoid protrusion of the mandible as a result of suboptimal correction. This leads to mandibular prognathism and an unsightly deformity known as the witch's chin. Controversy exists regarding the use of resorbable and nonresorbable materials for fixation. The former is biodegradable but may remain in situ with the potential to cause extrusion and foreign body reaction and also make the implant palpable under the soft skin of children. Nonresorbable materials, on the other hand, require a second surgery for removal and make future imaging unsafe for the patient in the event that it is required. Common complications include infection, nonunion, malunion and malocclusion, facial asymmetry due to disruption of growth of the mandible, interference with the eruption of permanent teeth, and dysfunction of the temporomandibular joint (TMJ). Treatment of these must be prolonged and involves orthodontic treatment, functional appliances and therapy, and the use of occlusal splints.

5.1.9 Dentition

Dentoalveolar trauma may involve the primary, mixed, or permanent dentition. The primary dentition is important for maintaining the space required for the growth of the permanent dentition so that the latter appears in a perfectly aligned manner. The permanent dentition is responsible for maintaining occlusion so that the intake and chewing of food are facilitated and also plays a part in ensuring a good external appearance and self-esteem, while contributing significantly to articulation of speech and vocal resonance.

Many classifications of dentoalveolar trauma are in use, but the simplest one probably is the one described the earliest by Sweet [3] and is as follows:

Class I—simple fracture of the crown with no exposure of dentin

Class II—parallel fracture of crown with exposure of minimal dentin

Class III—extensive fracture of crown with exposure of dentin but not the pulp

Class IV—extensive fracture of crown with exposure of dentin and also the pulp

Class V—complete fracture of crown with exposure of pulp

Class VI—fracture of tooth root with or without loss of crown structure

Class VII—total loss of tooth

The vitality and mobility of the tooth must be tested and the injury classified as stated above for each tooth involved in the trauma. Imaging of the affected tooth is done with the help of X-rays and appropriate antibiotics prescribed. It is important to know the immunization status of the child, and vaccines pending must be administered. Specific treatment options exist for each type of injury, which may be any of the following types:

(a) Infraction
(b) Uncomplicated enamel limited fracture
(c) Uncomplicated crown fracture
(d) Complicated crown fracture
(e) Uncomplicated crown-root fracture
(f) Complicated crown-root fracture
(g) Root fracture

Apart from the above, concussion, subluxation, lateral luxation, intrusion, extrusion, and avulsion injuries of the teeth, periodontal ligament, and soft tissues may also be seen.

5.1.10 Epistaxis

The nose and the nasal mucosa are extremely vascular structures. The chief vascular anastomoses may be found at the Kiesselbach's plexus or Little's area, which is where the terminal branches of all the blood vessels supplying the nasal septum meet. It is situated at the anteroinferior end of the septum and may be exposed to the external environment in cases of nasal septum deviation. Thus it is subjected to the drying effects of the air, and crusting may occur at this site, causing irritation and the tendency for nose picking. Digital trauma is therefore the most common cause of epistaxis from this area. Woodruff's plexus is a venous plexus situated near the posterior end of the inferior turbinate on the lateral wall of the nose, and elderly individuals with hypertension and atherosclerosis have a tendency to bleed from this region, especially as a result of vigorous nose blowing. The bleeding may be severe and difficult to control. At the posterior end of the middle turbinate on the lateral wall of the nose, the sphenopalatine artery is the major vessel to bleed. It is the terminal branch of the internal maxillary artery and is called the "artery of epistaxis" because of its large caliber and propensity to be torn, and this can lead to torrential hemorrhage as it exits from the sphenopalatine foramen and enters the nasal cavity.

Epistaxis is often a prominent symptom and sign of trauma to the head and face. It may occur even without serious injury to the bone and soft tissue elements in this region. It is also important to remember that traumatic epistaxis is usually limited by the impact and extent of injury unless medical illnesses such as high blood pressure, diabetes mellitus, or coagulopathies are also present. Thus, except in cases of severe facial or skull base injuries, the amount and duration of epistaxis are minimal to moderate, that is, it is usually self-limiting. Patients may even present with just a history of epistaxis following trauma but no active bleeding, and reassurance is all that is required in most instances. However, the presence of an external deformity or septal hematoma would warrant active surgical intervention.

Epistaxis may or may not accompany insertion of foreign bodies into the nose, but is more often encountered in attempts to remove the foreign body by inexperienced persons. Attention to technique, good illumination, and skill are of utmost importance. Inefficient removal may even allow the foreign body to slip deeper inside and lower down into the aerodigestive tract. Whenever such a situation is anticipated, the foreign body must be removed under general anesthesia taking care to first secure the airway. Endotracheal intubation may be avoided and the foreign body removed under mask ventilation and short anesthesia or sedation by putting the patient in slight head low position to avoid any slippage of the foreign body into the lower airway.

The role of hand dominance and blood groups has been studied in the etiopathology of epistaxis, but no large scale studies have been undertaken in this regard [4].

5.1.11 Cerebrospinal Fluid (CSF) Leaks

The incidence of CSF leak in fractures is highly variable, but most cases of CSF leak are traumatic in nature [5].

Cerebrospinal fluid (CSF) leaks of the anterior cranial base have been classified by Sakas into the following four types [6]:

1. I—cribriform
2. II—frontoethmoidal
3. III—lateral frontal
4. IV—complex

A fracture with a bony displacement of more than 1 cm is called large and that less than 1 cm is known as a small fracture. A large cribriform (type I) fracture is the most likely to result in infection (meningitis or encephalitis), whereas a small lateral frontal fracture is the least likely. Infection is also directly correlated with the compounded effects of rhinorrhea persisting for a longer time, a large amount of bony displacement at the fracture site, and distance from the midline, in that order.

Severe impact on the nose by a frontal impact can cause a complex and comminuted fracture of the nasal bones, which would then require treatment with a combination of open reduction and manipulation and fixation with wires, screws, or plates. The nasal septum may also be fractured in this type of injury, and deviation of the nasal bones and septum must be corrected together because "as the nose (nasal bone) goes, so goes the septum." If the ethmoid complex is injured, the septum is again liable to be involved and must be addressed. There is the added problem of a cerebrospinal fluid leak requiring repair of the same and consolidation of the skull base.

Cerebrospinal fluid (CSF) rhinorrhea may occur by several mechanisms. The most common is trauma to the skull base as is seen in head injuries and motor vehicle accidents. The size of the defect can range from small to large. The initial symptom is bleeding from the nose or epistaxis, and a close check must be made for the halo sign or handkerchief test. The patient's clothes or bed linen must be examined. The halo sign refers to the appearance of a clear zone outside the area of the bloodstain because the presence of CSF, which has a lower density, allows the stain to advance beyond the distance covered by blood, which has a higher density. Though this is a useful bedside test, it is not very reliable or foolproof, and many a time, CSF is missed in the initial days of a head injury. CSF leak may also occur through the nose in the absence of epistaxis, and in such cases, it is fluid that escapes via the auditory tube following a temporal bone fracture, and such a leak is known as CSF otorhinorrhea.

A CSF leak may be obvious in cases of acute trauma or occult in cases of old and forgotten trauma masquerading as attacks of bacterial meningitis. Thus any patient with meningitis must be investigated for possible recent or old trauma in the absence of the usual risk factors. The site of leak may be in the temporal bone as well in which case the leak would manifest as a CSF otorhinorrhea if the tympanic membrane (TM) is intact or a CSF otorrhea if the TM is ruptured.

The other most common mechanism of a CSF leak in recent times is iatrogenic trauma. This is encountered in endoscopic surgery for the paranasal sinuses and skull base. Prior to the endoscopic era also, CSF leaks were common during procedures such as septal surgery and intranasal polypectomy owing to poor technique and uncontrolled removal of tissue. Microdebrider-assisted endoscopic surgeries also tend to cause mucosal avulsions and increase the chances of not only CSF leak but injury to the anterior ethmoidal and internal carotid arteries and the optic nerve. Unfavorable configurations of the anterior skull base, such as a Keros type 2 or 3, greatly increase the potential for iatrogenic CSF leaks.

Apart from trauma, the other common mechanism is congenital defects, but they shall not be discussed here, except for the fact that a congenital defect or weakness in the skull base makes it even more vulnerable to a traumatic insult.

CSF leaks may follow a transsphenoidal hypophysectomy, in which case it is not only iatrogenic but an integral step of the surgery. Large leaks must be repaired using bone, cartilage, fat, mucosa, fascia lata, and tissue glue, with various combinations.

5.2   Clinical Implications

5.2.1   Treatment Planning

The demographics of trauma have been studied in different settings but quite a few similarities become evident. One is that in the elderly, falls and elder abuse constitute the main causes. At the opposite age extreme, which is in children, falls and accidental insertion of foreign bodies make up the chief etiologies. In the active middle years, interpersonal violence and motor vehicle accidents are the principal culprits. Males are more commonly affected in general except in domestic violence or physical assault against spouses, in which case women are more affected. Alcohol use and abuse are both positively correlated to the frequency and cause of trauma in middle-aged males, as would be expected in interpersonal violence and motor vehicle accidents.

Trauma to the facial skeleton may also have different effects that vary according to the patient's age. For example, greenstick fractures are common in children and young adults as the bones are very elastic, and only one cortex suffers a break while the other is intact. This type of fracture results in soft tissue contusion, but deformity is not marked as bone fragments are not much displaced from each other. On the other hand, even low-impact trauma is capable of shattering the bone in elderly patients, especially women, as they tend to have osteoporosis. Comminuted fractures with deformity are commonly seen though the extent of injury may not be readily apparent due to the relative laxity of the overlying skin.

Facial reconstruction techniques were first described by the pioneering French facial plastic and reconstructive surgeon Paul Tessier who undertook the same for the correction of congenital deformities in children. These provided daring approaches and wider access with carefully planned incisions and methods of reconstruction using autologous grafts to restore form and function to the maximum extent possible. As the head and neck region houses organs responsible for not only external appearance but also the special senses, respiration, swallowing, voicing, and chewing food, optimal management is crucial if quality of life is to be maintained. Facial fractures not only cause cosmetic deformity but also functional impairment and life-threatening damage if the internal organs such as the globe of the eye, optic nerve, brain, skull base, lacrimal apparatus, and infraorbital nerve are involved. The implications of injury in the cranial cavity and skull base, and to the orbit, infraorbital nerve, and inferior alveolar nerve, are enormous.

The workup of the trauma patient and planning treatment of the injuries must take into account all of the above aspects.

5.2.2 Investigations

The clinical assessment of facial trauma may be confounded by the presence of dressings and bandages and the endotracheal and nasogastric tubes that are often inserted during the management of the patient. These may also make identification of impacted foreign bodies difficult and may result in not identifying pieces of missing tissue.

5.2.3 Imaging

Plain X-rays are not useful at all in planning the management of the patient and may be taken only for medicolegal (MLC) purposes in the case of nasal bone fractures (Fig. 5.1).

Imaging for facial trauma may be done with fan beam CT or cone beam CT. Cone beam CT provides better definition and less radiation exposure. Digital volume technology (DVT) is an advanced mode employed in CT scanning. Both intraoperative and postoperative CT may be taken; the former allows real-time assessment of fracture reduction and intraoperative adjustments. Skull base fractures can be better managed using computer navigation. Three-dimensional (3D) CT imaging is especially useful in facial fractures for providing accurate definition of bony structures and the type of management required. Radiation exposure due to CT imaging is a

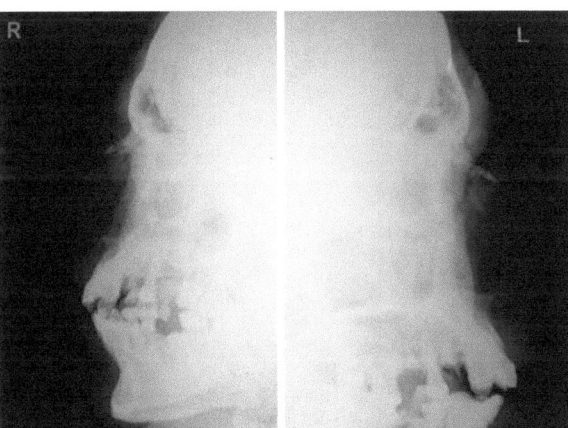

Fig. 5.1 X-ray nasal bones showing fracture

limiting factor and advanced techniques such as 3D CT and high-resolution CT (HRCT) render high doses of radiation to the patient, roughly equivalent to 2.0 millisieverts, that is, equivalent to 20 or greater plain chest X-rays at the minimum. The harmful effects of radiation are commonly manifested as premature cataract, and it is believed that the above level of radiation exposure is enough to lead to this complication. Thus, even though CT imaging forms an integral part of the management of trauma, due care should be exercised and radiation exposure minimized by thorough clinical evaluation and only resorting to imaging that is absolutely essential.

A coronal CT scan is useful for delineation of the orbital and maxillary walls, the ethmoids and sphenoid, and the pterygoid plates and palate.

CT imaging with axial and coronal cuts would show up not only fractures and soft tissue injuries but also help to decide if an endoscopic repair is possible. The contours of the frontal sinuses, orbital walls, nasolacrimal duct (NLD), and optic canal can be seen clearly on the bone windows of the CT scan (Figs. 5.2, 5.3, 5.4, 5.5, 5.6, and 5.7).

In addition to the axial and coronal CT cuts, reformatted parasagittal cuts in the posteromedial to anterolateral direction may be constructed for better definition of the optic canal in order to rule out optic nerve injury. This reconstruction in the sagittal plane, and three-dimensional (3D) reconstruction for better definition of the facial skeleton for surgical planning, is possible only if the axial cuts are at least 1.5 mm apart and not more. Wider cuts tend to produce more artifacts and may confuse the clinical assessment.

Imaging for maxillofacial trauma includes 3D CT reconstructions that would help to direct surgical treatment. Whether closed reduction would suffice or open reduction with internal fixation (ORIF) is required can be judged based on the 3D CT because it is able to define exact planes of displacement of the bony elements of the facial skeleton.

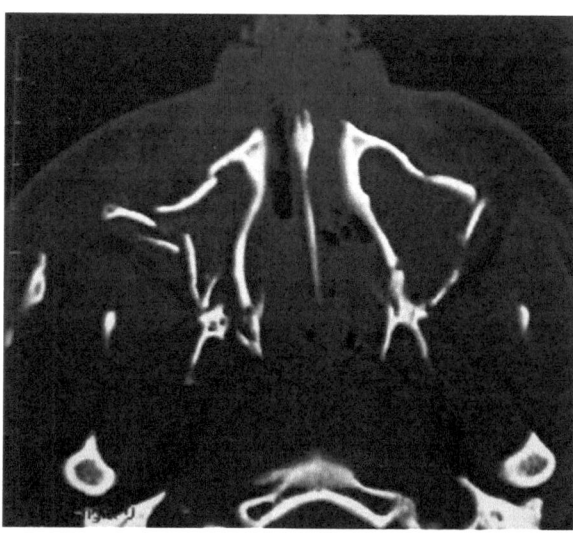

Fig. 5.2 CT axial view showing fracture maxilla

Fig. 5.3 CT paranasal sinuses showing multiple fractures

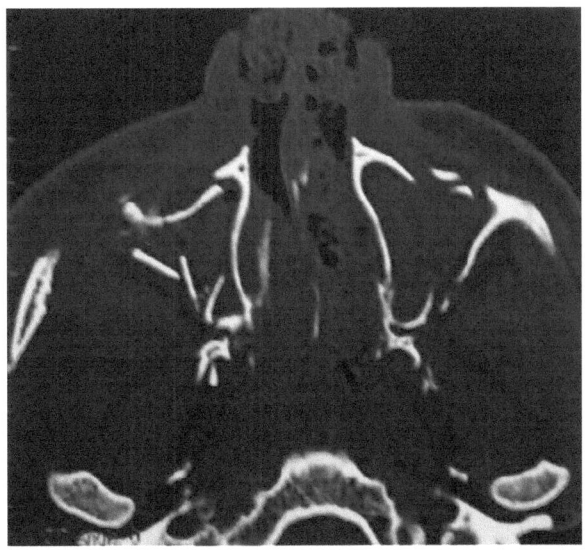

Fig. 5.4 CT PNS fine cuts showing extent of fractures

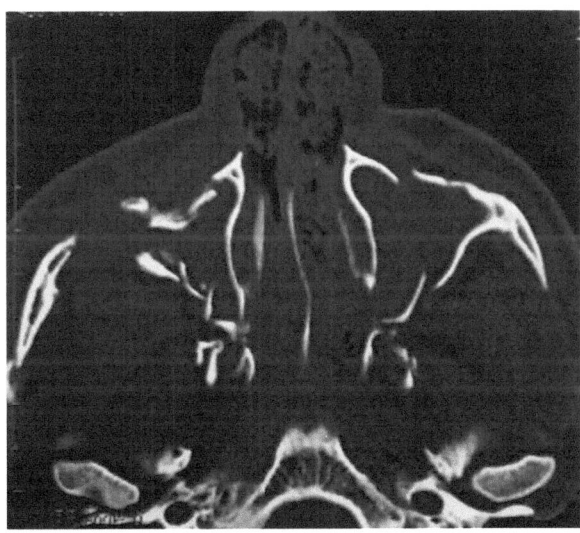

Following surgical treatment, further imaging is generally not required to assess the completeness or correctness of the repair as long as it has been executed along expected lines. If difficulty is encountered or the repair has failed, the imaging may be repeated using 3D CT. Plain X-rays do not serve any purpose in this regard and not only provide a false sense of security but also increase the radiation exposure [7].

CT scanning during the surgical repair or use of a C-arm is a useful adjunct for fine-tuning the outcome of the procedure. It is also useful for the purpose of teaching and training of residents in trauma surgery, especially when dealing with multiple or complex maxillofacial trauma [8].

Fig. 5.5 CT PNS axial
view with soft tissue injury

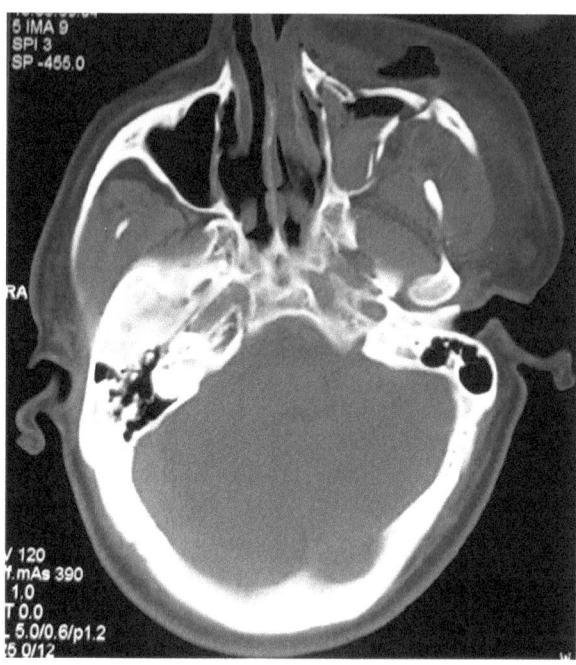

Fig. 5.6 CT PNS coronal
view with soft tissue injury

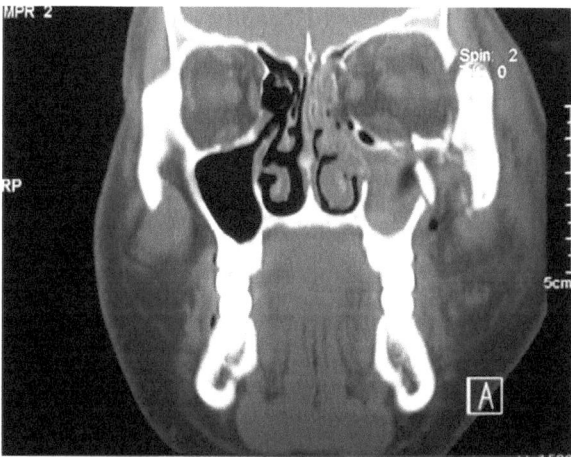

CT scan is an important tool for the diagnosis and management of complex maxillofacial trauma, especially since the same modality may be used for other related trauma such as head and orthopedic trauma.

Imaging in the form of HRCT of the paranasal sinuses and skull base using axial and coronal cuts, and if necessary sagittal reformatted sections, is highly useful in the detection and location of small cerebrospinal fluid (CSF) leaks which are not actively or obviously discharging [9]. CT cisternography in addition to this may provide evidence of brain herniation and CSF leak (Figs. 5.8, 5.9, 5.10, 5.11, and 5.12).

Fig. 5.7 CT PNS sagittal
cuts with soft tissue injury

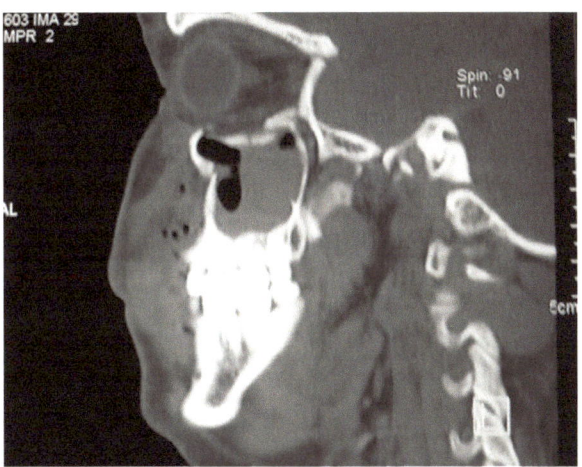

Fig. 5.8 CT
cisternography coronal
view; early phase

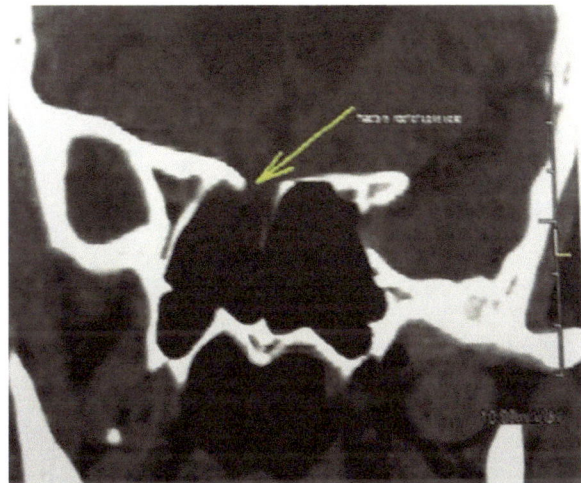

Fig. 5.9 CT
cisternography coronal
view; late phase

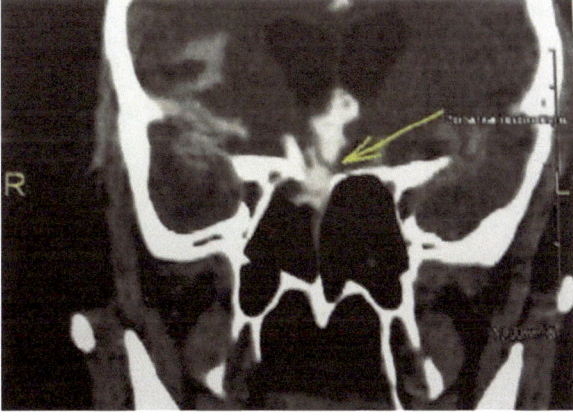

Fig. 5.10 CT
cisternography axial view

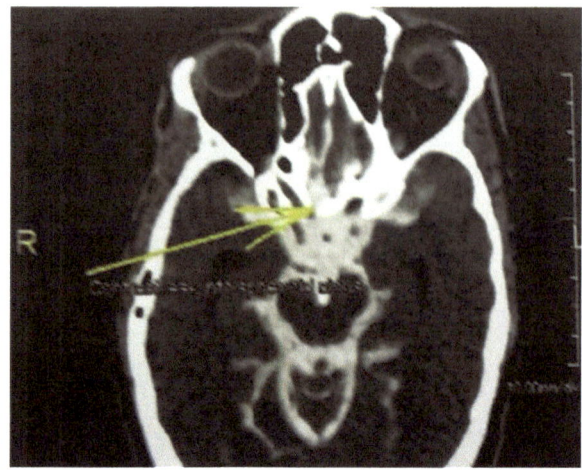

Fig. 5.11 CT
cisternography sagittal
view; early phase

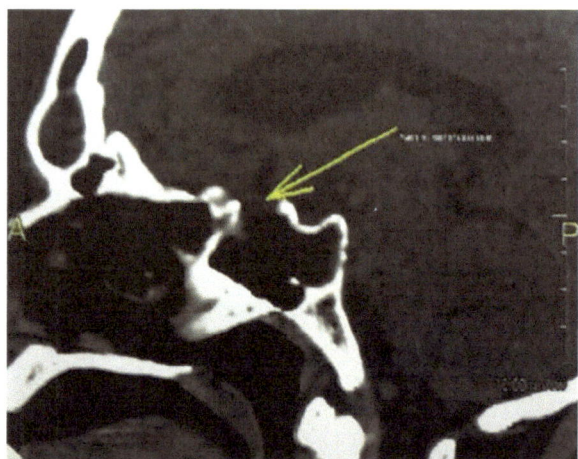

Fig. 5.12 CT
cisternography sagittal
view; late phase

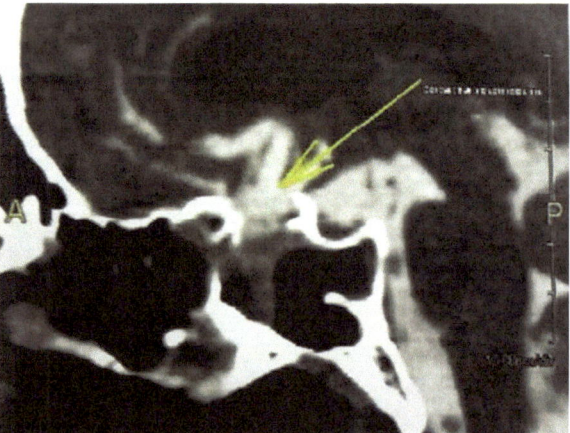

Other methods of investigation include CT metrizamide scan, CT with MRI, ventriculography, and fluorescein angiography. Imaging in the form of plain CT scan, along with MRI, is a noninvasive method to detect the presence of a leak. The CT scan defines the bone disruption, while MRI reveals brain tissue herniation in the T1-weighted images and presence of CSF in the T2-weighted images. Earlier modalities of imaging such as CT cisternography are also useful and employ a contrast agent injected intrathecally. A CT metrizamide scan may also be done using an intravenously injected contrast.

5.2.4   Biochemistry

The presence or absence of cerebrospinal fluid (CSF) may be determined on the basis of the beta-2 transferrin test, which is highly sensitive (99%) and specific. However, at least 0.1 ml of fluid is required, which is difficult to obtain in cases where the leak is small, and the drainage is little and occurring intermittently during periods of strain. Also, a few days are required for assay of this substance and the management has to be deferred accordingly. Other substances may also be looked for, such as beta-trace protein (BTP), glucose, and electrolytes, but these are nonspecific and may be found in nasal secretions, perilymph, and aqueous humor. The target or halo sign, though popular, is sometimes unreliable and cannot be assumed as conclusive evidence of a cerebrospinal fluid (CSF) leak.

5.2.5   Other Tests

Last but not least, a leak may be detected by direct visualization on table using fluorescein dye which has been introduced intrathecally. This is described further in this chapter.

5.2.6   Treatment Procedure

The procedural treatment for different types of injuries to the nose and facial skeleton is herewith described individually.

5.2.7   Nasal Septum and Nasal Bones

Treatment for nasal trauma due to birth molding may be carried out immediately after birth, though this is not commonly done. Application of forceps or suction is an added risk for such trauma. If the injury is severe in nature, the baby may present with snuffles or respiratory distress due to the nasal mucosal congestion and/or septal hematoma. By introducing a pair of prongs into the nasal cavities and applying sustained pressure over the nasal floor, it is possible to reduce the septal cartilage fracture and deviation. Hematomas, if present, can be aspirated and soft splints given to support the reduction. If left untreated at birth, such injuries would present in early childhood with severe nasal obstruction, at which time a guarded septoplasty can be carried out. Definitive correction of the nasal septum is ideally done after 18 years of age when the growth of the facial skeleton is completed.

A septal hematoma is common after a septal fracture as the blood collects under the mucoperichondrium of the nasal septum. Such an occurrence is more likely in children and young adults as well as women, who have softer and more elastic tissues and suffer more greenstick fractures as a result of the same.

The presence of a hematoma leads to aseptic necrosis of the septal cartilage as its blood supply from the mucosa is cut off. Thus a hematoma must be treated expediently by incision and drainage and a snug anterior nasal packing to provide tamponade of the mucosa and prevent re-accumulation of the blood. A septal hematoma may also predispose to infection and abscess formation, both of which may be treated with intravenous antibiotics after first relieving the purulent exudates. The risk of complications such as cavernous sinus thrombosis and orbital or frontal lobe abscess remains high in these patients.

A nasal septal perforation may also result from loss of septal cartilage at the time of injury or aseptic necrosis at a later date due to a neglected septal hematoma. It may also be the result of aggressive treatment of bleeding from Little's area by chemical or electrical cauterization. If anteriorly sited, it produces an annoying whistling sound on respiration and would need to be repaired using a mucosal flap designed from the surrounding nasal mucosa. If large, it causes crusting and a flapping septum. Repair is more difficult in these cases and may be suitably managed with the help of silastic buttons, obturators, or prostheses.

Deformity caused by neglected trauma, if more than 3 weeks in duration, must be treated with a mix and match of septorhinoplasty and cosmetic facial surgery.

Complications such as septal hematoma, abscess, and perforation may also be iatrogenic in nature if suitable care and meticulous technique in the treatment of either primary nasal trauma or nontraumatic disorders such as correction of septal or turbinate problems and neoplastic lesions are not carried out.

Minor fractures of the nasal bones without displacement and causing no other deformity apart from the accompanying edema and contusion require only conservative management. If there is a nosebleed, it may be managed with decongestant drops or gentle anterior nasal packing to provide a sort of splintage, which may be removed after 24–72 h.

A more serious degree of injury may cause some displacement of the nasal bones, which can then be reduced into position and alignment by closed manipulation using a pair of Walsham's forceps. These are sturdy and designed in a manner to both provide a strong grip for the nasal bone as well as minimize injury to the overlying skin as the manual reduction is carried out. Asch's forceps is a similar kind of forceps used for the reduction of a septal fracture. It has a space between the jaws to avoid crushing of the nasal septal cartilage.

Clinical photographs and documentation for nasal bone fractures are extremely important both from the point of view of optimal correction and patient satisfaction and also for medicolegal purposes (Figs. 5.13, 5.14, 5.15, 5.16, 5.17, and 5.18).

Even compound injuries with trauma to the facial skin and soft tissues must be similarly documented (Figs. 5.19 and 5.20).

Wherever possible, comparison with pre-injury photographs is desirable so as to avoid unrealistic expectations. Other injuries such as internal mucosal injuries may also be photographed for academic and medicolegal purposes (Fig. 5.21).

Fig. 5.13 Fracture nasal bones; front view

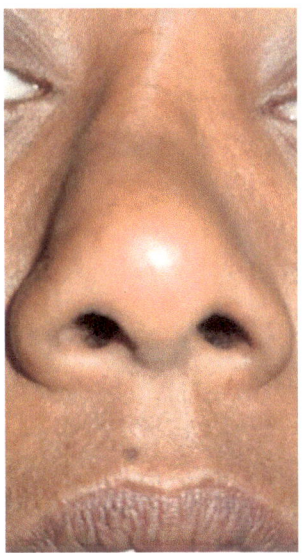

Fig. 5.14 Fracture nasal bones; tip view

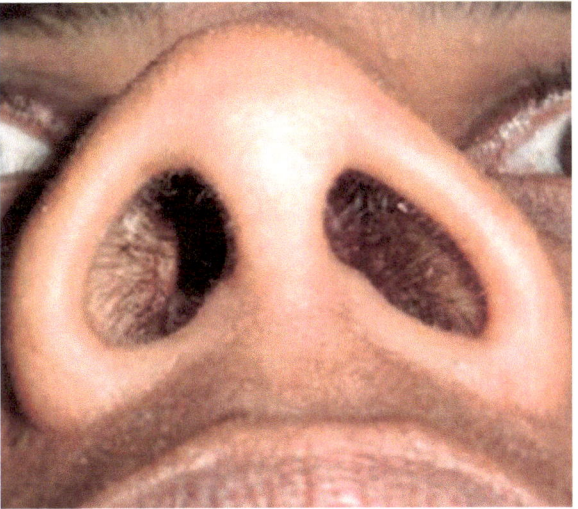

Fig. 5.15 Fracture nasal
bones; right lateral view

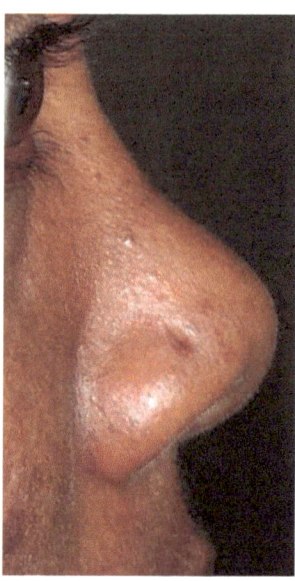

Fig. 5.16 Fracture nasal
bones; left lateral view

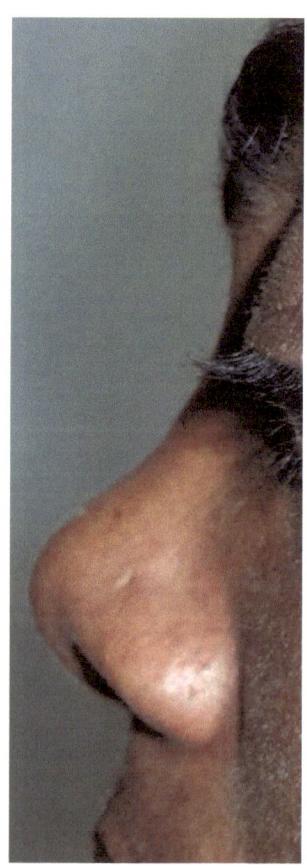

Fig. 5.17 Fracture nasal bones; right lateral oblique view

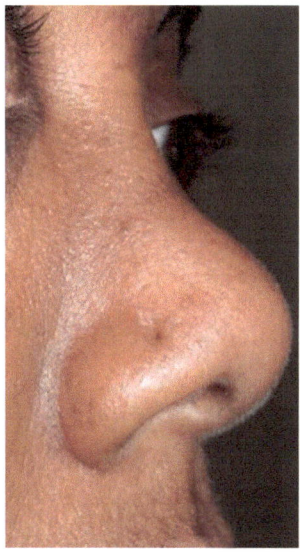

Fig. 5.18 Fracture nasal bones; left lateral oblique view

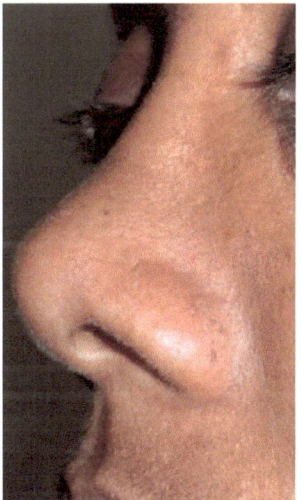

5.2.8   Epistaxis

In severe cases of traumatic epistaxis, it is imperative to control blood loss. Most centers adopt nasal packing—anterior, posterior, or both—in order to provide tamponade to the nasal mucosa and prevent further blood loss. Tamponade causes the bleeding vessel or site to be mechanically compressed or to undergo spasm but is not helpful in localizing the actual site of bleeding. Before undertaking nasal packing, the presence of a cerebrospinal fluid leak should be ruled out as far as possible. This is because the presence of a foreign body such as a nasal pack predisposes to

Fig. 5.19 Facial compound wound with split nose

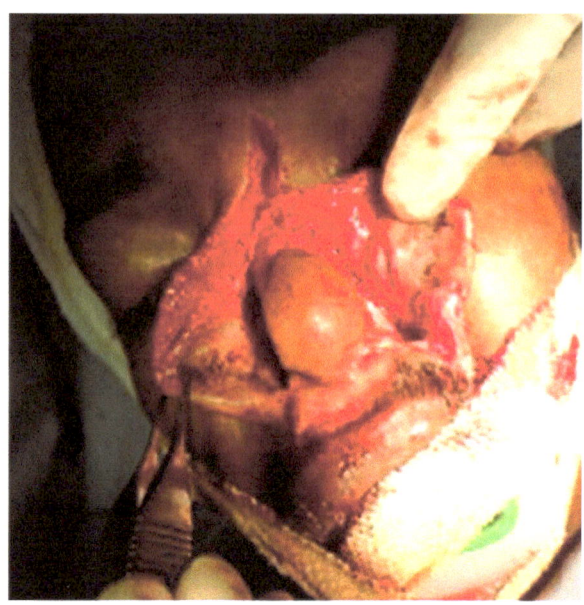

Fig. 5.20 Split nose sutured

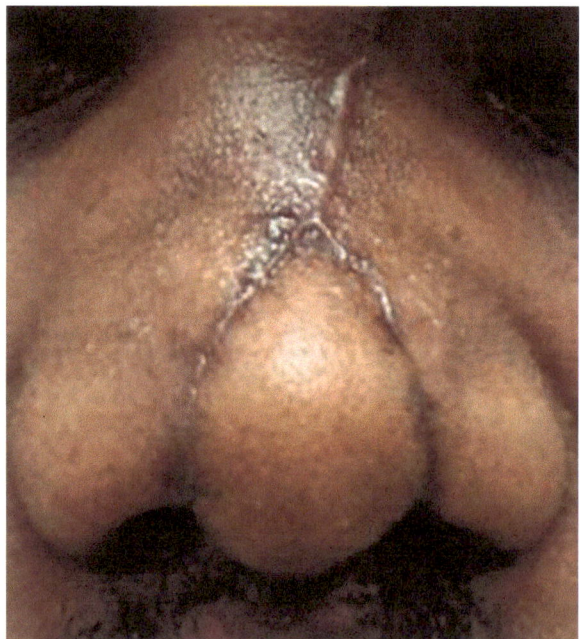

Fig. 5.21 Mucosal
injury—hematoma tongue

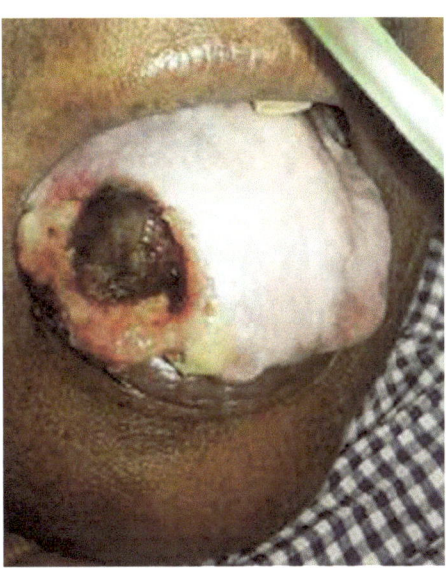

infection and could also lead to intracranial complications such as meningitis and
brain abscess. Although presterilized and prepackaged packs such as Merocel are
now widely available, steam-sterilized roller gauze packs are still used in many
parts of the world, especially in developing countries and underserved areas. The
risk of infection is high in the presence of nasal packs, and antibiotics in either oral
or parenteral form are always recommended.

Nasal packing causes significant discomfort to the patient with symptoms such
as headache, dryness of the mouth, watering of the eyes, and blood-stained discharge through the pack engorged with nasal secretions. In many centers, therefore, nasal packing is not the preferred mode of management of epistaxis. In less
serious cases, head end elevation, nasal decongestant drops, antifibrinolytic agents
such as tranexamic acid, and medications to control elevated blood pressure or
medical conditions if any, may be adopted. In persistent epistaxis, the options
include embolization and transnasal endoscopic sphenopalatine artery ligation
(TESPAL). Embolization of the sphenopalatine artery on one or both sides may be
done for traumatic epistaxis without any significant side effects [10]. Embolization
is carried out through the transfemoral route using the Seldinger technique
(Figs. 5.22 and 5.23).

Although nasal packing could be done as an emergency procedure in cases
selected for the above procedures, there exist alternative and less invasive ways to
reduce the blood loss through the nose in order to facilitate the same. One is the use
of hypotensive anesthesia and modified Moffat's solution as used in endoscopic
sinus surgeries (ESS). The other is by administering a greater palatine artery block
through the greater palatine foramen located over the palate using an intraoral
approach. Both these methods require the use of a state-of-the-art endoscopic suite
and expert staffing, and of course, the patient's general condition should allow the

Fig. 5.22 Sphenopalatine embolization—catheter in place

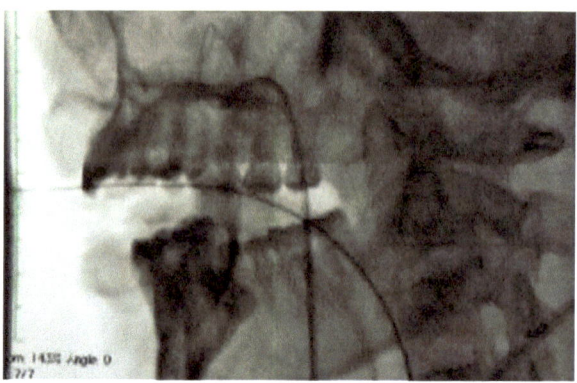

Fig. 5.23 Sphenopalatine embolization done

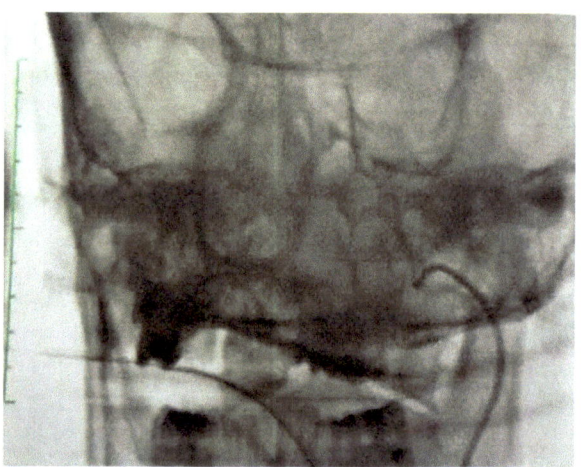

same. The presence of severe trismus due to complex facial fractures would preclude the use of these techniques.

In cases where nasal packing has already been done, further anxiety awaits both doctor and patient at the time of removal of the pack. The pack may be removed in 24–72 h depending on the case and the propensity to bleed again. Pack removal is as traumatic for the patient as is its insertion and due care must be exercised during both the steps. A well-lubricated pack and proper technique are essential, and otolaryngologists are suitably trained in these principles. Lubrication with medications such as antibiotic creams and bismuth iodoform paraffin paste (BIPP) is to be done at the time of pack insertion, and agents such as liquid paraffin may be used during the removal of the same pack. It is better to start instilling the liquid paraffin drops using a dropper or syringe at least 2 h before the removal of the pack in ideal circumstances but also at the time of the actual procedure of removal using more quantities of the solution.

Packs lubricated with BIPP may be kept in situ for up to 5 days without significant risk of infection. This is because bismuth is a chelating agent and has a hygroscopic action on the mucosa, thus reducing mucosal edema and inflammation. The iodine in the preparation acts as an antiseptic, while the paraffin paste provides an emollient action, making BIPP the optimal pack to use, probably next only to or even better than the Merocel packs. However it is cumbersome to prepare, and the raw ingredients are not easily available in many regions, making it less popular.

Bleeding during pack removal can be managed in the same way as has been described above in the methods to avoid nasal packing using simple measures. It is usually not necessary to reinsert another nasal pack, but a little patience and perseverance are needed. Junior staff in busy practices often tend to forget this and proceed to repacking, which is not only extremely traumatic for the patient but is also scientifically unsound and a waste of resources.

5.2.9   Frontal Sinus

When dealing with fractures of the frontal sinus, it is crucial to bear in mind the twin requirements of preservation of structural form and physiological function and the avoidance of complications. The different routes by which surgical access can be gained are the Lynch-Howarth, subciliary, transconjunctival, gingivobuccal, lateral rhinotomy, and midfacial degloving approaches if open surgery is being contemplated or the transnasal endoscopic approach. Fixation may be done by wiring and plating, using a titanium mesh, implant or prosthesis, or by a regional or free tissue transfer.

Frontal sinus fractures may be managed conservatively or surgically, with procedures such as open reduction and internal fixation (ORIF), obliteration of the sinus, or cranialization of the sinus. ORIF is usually done for limited fractures involving the anterior table of the frontal sinus bone, whereas obliteration must be done when there is extensive trauma with gross devitalization of the frontal sinus mucosa and injury in the area of the frontal outflow tract. Autologous fat is commonly used to fill the sinus in an obliteration procedure. Cranialization, on the other hand, is undertaken for disruption of the posterior table of the frontal sinus bone and herniation of brain or meninges into the sinus. In this procedure, the posterior table and sinus mucosa are removed, the frontal outflow tract obliterated, and the inner lining of the frontal sinus replaced with periosteum and allowed to be in contiguity with the intracranial cavity. Frontal sinus injury may manifest in long-term symptoms, and late complications in the form of cellulitis, meningitis, and osteomyelitis have been known to appear even up to 25 years.

Frontal sinus fractures were traditionally repaired using open surgical approaches. Fractures of the posterior plate of the frontal bone and sinus were fixed with the cavity of the sinus made continuous with the intracranial cavity after complete removal of any remnants of frontal sinus mucosa. This was known as cranialization. Alternatively, fractures of the anterior table were treated with complete exenteration of the frontal sinus contents and repair using soft tissue and bone graft in order to restore cosmetic appearance of the face. This procedure was called obliteration of the frontal sinus.

Both cranialization and obliteration are associated with considerable morbidity and loss of sinus function [11], and with the advent of the rigid nasal endoscope, a completely endoscopic or partial (conservative) endoscopic approach has gained popularity, improving both functional and esthetic outcomes [12].

5.2.10 Cerebrospinal Fluid (CSF) Leak

Approximately 10–50% of cases of facial, frontal bone and frontal sinus, and anterior skull base trauma may result in a cerebrospinal fluid (CSF) leak. Conversely, most cases of cerebrospinal fluid (CSF) leaks are due to trauma, and a small number may be due to congenital and developmental causes and skull base tumors. The risk of meningitis is high in cerebrospinal fluid (CSF) leaks, and the incidence varies as described according to the Sakas classification mentioned above.

In general, traumatic leaks if small tend to close spontaneously with minimal intervention and long-term sequelae. If medium, they respond favorably to conservative measures like head high position with the head turned to the side opposite the leak, avoidance of straining or sneezing, and drugs like acetazolamide (Diamox) to decrease the production of CSF. Larger leaks need to be treated with surgery—either endoscopic or open—with or without a CSF diversion procedure like lumbar drain or ventriculoperitoneal shunt.

Fractures of the anterior cranial base at the region of the cribriform plate rarely undergo spontaneous closure and require surgical management. The good news is that most of these may be approached nasally with an endoscope and thus avoid the many sequelae seen in the case of open procedures such as a frontal craniotomy or bicoronal approach/bifrontal craniofacial resection.

Intrathecal fluorescein uses 0.1 ml of a concentration of 5–10% fluorescein diluted in 10 ml of CSF and is seen as a green fluorescence in the nasal mucosa at the site of the leak. It is not without its side effects, some of which are minor, for example tinnitus, headache, nausea, vomiting, and confusion, and the others major, including coma, seizures, pulmonary edema, and even death. Only conservative management is adequate for most of the leaks caused by trauma, and almost 70–85% close this way within a few weeks. If left untreated, anywhere from 7 to 70% of leaks would result in meningitis. Figures vary due to differences in reporting.

The majority of CSF leaks (about 70%) close with conservative management, which may consist of head end elevation, use of carbonic anhydrase inhibitors, avoidance of straining and nose blowing, and diversion of CSF with the use of a lumbar drain or ventriculostomy [13]. Controlled positive pressure with the use of straws, incentive spirometers, and Valsalva maneuver is also beneficial in the closure of small leaks. This may be undertaken when a history of meningitis is present but no fluid is found on straining. Repair of such leaks must be done as they might have become true epithelialized fistulous tracts, and the repair must be done in the same fashion as primary repair. Pneumococcal vaccine may be given as an adjunctive treatment.

The leaks arising from the sphenoid, cribriform, or ethmoid roof may all be repaired using an endoscopic extracranial approach, with a high rate of success [14]. Control of bleeding is very important in CSF leak closure as intracranial bleeding predisposes to hypoxic brain injury [15].

Although it makes intuitive sense to administer prophylactic antibiotics when a cerebrospinal fluid (CSF) leak is detected, such practice has not been proved to provide substantial benefit as far as prevention of meningitis is concerned [16]. If conservative measures directed at reducing CSF pressure to aid spontaneous closure of the leak fail within a reasonable period of time, then a surgical closure of the defect is recommended as early as possible. Nowadays most CSF leaks situated in the cribriform area can be repaired using the endoscopic approach. Sphenoid sinus leaks are less amenable to endoscopic repair except in cases of iatrogenic defects caused during pituitary surgery, in which case the defect is mostly central in location and more easily accessible through the same route as employed for tumor excision. Traumatic leaks involving the lateral wall of the sphenoid are best managed with an open approach or an endoscopic transpterygoid approach after ligation of the sphenopalatine artery. Otherwise only large defects in the posterior aspect of the anterior skull base require an open route such as craniotomy or anterior craniofacial approach, and such defects are more commonly encountered in spontaneous leaks due to congenital malformations or following tumor resection and are not relevant to the management of traumatic leaks.

The repair of cerebrospinal fluid leaks may be done by an inlay or onlay method using autologous or homologous fascia, fat, cartilage, pericranium, and finally bone, usually in that sequence. Small leaks could be sealed with a "bath plug" using fat, but this is not recommended for larger defects, for which a full and layered repair should be done. The repair is done in layers to provide an airtight seal, and the use of a lumbar drain for diversion of CSF is not absolutely necessary. Both pediatric and adult traumatic leaks may be treated by endoscopic closure of the defect provided the site of leak is favorable for the endoscopic approach. A fascia lata graft taken from the lateral aspect of the thigh provides adequate tissue for the repair of large defects. Local tissue from the nose, such as nasal septal perichondrium or cartilage, and turbinate mucosa taken either as free or rotated grafts may be used for smaller defects, but the fascia lata graft gives better results.

5.2.11 Frontal Sinus Outflow Tract

Frontal sinus fractures commonly involve the frontal sinus outflow tract, and involvement of this area results in a high risk of stenosis. Primary repair can be undertaken in this area if detected in time, but more often the consequence of stenosis of the frontal outflow tract is the late development of frontal and frontoethmoidal mucoceles. Most mucoceles, except large ones in the lateral reaches of the frontal sinus, are amenable to an endoscopic approach for undertaking excision and repair. The Draf IIa, IIb, and III (modified Lothrop) procedures may all be undertaken for the treatment of traumatic mucoceles, but the Draf IIb procedure is most commonly associated with the risk of restenosis [17].

Open approaches such as the osteoplastic flap repair are highly effective but are associated with a recurrence rate of about 25%, and in recent times, modifications of this have been used [18]. Hydroxyapatite may be used for contouring the bony repair and improving appearance.

Treatment of frontal sinus fractures is fraught with unpredictable outcomes in some cases, and complications have been seen as late as 25 years following the initial injury [19].

To ensure good appearance and proper function, and to avoid poor outcomes including pain and discomfort as well as the risk of late complications such as sinusitis and chronic dacryocystitis, systematic fixation of the fractured segments with plates and screws must be done after proper reduction and realignment in order to minimize callus, infection, and shifting of fragments [20].

5.2.12 Zygoma and Maxilla

Each type of zygomaticomaxillary complex (ZMC) fracture should be reduced, aligned properly, and fixed so that the least amount of plating and disruption of soft tissue is involved [21]. The management is by maxilla-mandibular fixation (MMF), repair of the orbital blowout fracture, nasolacrimal duct (NLD) and optic canal injuries if any, and providing skin and soft tissue cover.

Optimal methods include a miniplate and screw fixation at the zygomaticomaxillary (ZM) buttress, zygomatic-frontal (ZF) suture, inferior orbital rim, or zygomatic arch as the case may be.

If there is no significant deformity or nerve injury, conservative management would suffice. Otherwise, closed reduction through a temporal incision may be attempted, failing which ORIF may be carried out. Dissection in the subcutaneous plane in an inferior direction helps to mobilize the fracture fragments, which may then be gently manipulated into position, confirmed by a "clicking" sound and feel. Packing of the maxillary sinus must be done to maintain reduction, fixation, and immobilization.

5.2.13 Mandible and Temporomandibular Joint (TMJ)

There is wide variability in treatment techniques depending on individual preferences of the operating surgeon, but concern for the surrounding vital structures remains paramount [22].

When treating difficult midfacial fractures, the mandible, if intact, can be used as a stable base, and the maxillary dentition can be made to rest on this. This also helps to restore dental occlusion and allows restoration of the facial contour in a bottom-to-top fashion [23].

In recent times, the endoscopic approach has become popular with many surgeons, but the availability of proper endoscopic equipment is imperative [24]. If an external approach is contemplated, it is essential to ensure stability of the cervical spine so that a cervical collar, if present, may be safely removed.

After the temporomandibular joint (TMJ) and the fractured condyle has been exposed, the dissection is carried anteriorly until the articular eminence and entire TMJ capsule are seen clearly. At this stage the mandible can be opened and closed so that both visualization and palpation may be done for confirmation. Dissection then proceeds inferiorly along with retraction so that the subcondylar region is reached and fixation can be done [25].

Complications, especially in children, include damage to the inferior alveolar nerve following screw placement into the mandibular canal, thus injuring the nerve [26]. Plating may be done using metal or polydioxanone (PDS), which is biodegradable.

The mandible is the strongest in the teeth-bearing regions, and the condyles and symphysis menti are relatively weaker. Anterior overjet and anterior overbite must be identified and corrected promptly to prevent malocclusion.

Up to 20–60% of fractures of the mandible include the condyle fractures and are therefore the most common. Though individual preferences vary, surgical correction by either the open or closed method may be done, and both give similar results. The goal is to restore normal occlusion and baseline jaw biomechanics so that chewing and cosmesis are not affected. In this regard, it is worthwhile remembering that fractures of both condyles, if present simultaneously, are better treated by open surgical techniques as closed reduction does not provide good results.

While considering open surgery, attention must be directed toward the general condition of the patient and presence of comorbid conditions. Maxilla-mandibular fixation is a popular open surgical option, but more and more surgeons prefer the endoscopic approach for the reduction of mandibular fractures. This is especially useful if the fracture is intracapsular or involves the neck of the mandible. The endoscopic approach also avoids prolonged maxilla-mandibular fixation and reduces the risk of ankylosis of the jaw, which is significant if immobilization of the jaw exceeds a week to 10 days. Also, nonerupted teeth may be injured in open approaches using intermaxillary fixation screws. Both wiring and elastic bands may be suitably employed for fixation, and the latter are easier to remove in an emergency situation such as airway obstruction but cannot be used in patients who are agitated, reluctant, or not compliant.

The open approach also mandates removal of the cervical collar if any, so it is crucial to ensure that the cervical spine is not involved. General anesthesia for reduction is preferred using nasotracheal intubation so that jaw reduction and alignment are optimized.

The various incisions used for the treatment of mandibular fractures are the submandibular or Risdon incision and the preauricular and retromandibular incisions, all of which pose considerable risk to the facial nerve. In contrast, the intraoral approach, though not providing a wide exposure, protects the facial nerve and avoids an externally visible scar. Thus it is easy to understand why the endoscopic route is becoming more and more popular nowadays. Better optical and computer technology ensure a minimally invasive, safe, and effective approach for these fractures. The usual complications are bleeding, swelling or bruising, trismus and pain, damage to the teeth or bone, and injury to the infraorbital and inferior alveolar nerves. Serious complications include airway obstruction due to displacement of reduction, hematoma, edema, or aspiration of a tooth or foreign body. In the immediate postoperative period, complications such as cellulitis and abscess, dehiscence of the wound, and loosening of teeth, implants, or prostheses may occur and must be promptly identified and managed. Late complications include an unsightly scar, parotid fistula, nonunion, malunion, ankylosis of the jaw, chronic osteomyelitis of the mandible, resorption of the mandibular condyle, and interference with the growth of the facial skeleton.

5.2.14 Dentition

Injury to the teeth may involve the tooth proper (crown, root, enamel, dentine, and pulp), the periodontal ligament, and the alveolar bone socket in which the tooth is housed. The incisors and premolars are the most liable to injury. Loose fragments of teeth or missing teeth should be actively searched for in the surrounding tissues, gastrointestinal tract and airway, and replanted or removed. CT imaging may be required to find missing teeth. Fractures with displacement may be simply splinted with the help of interdental wiring until healing takes place in about 2 weeks. Chipping of the enamel may be treated with capping using a variety of materials. Complex or severe fractures, impaction, laceration of the gingiva with tears of the periodontal ligament, and injury to the tooth pulp require thorough cleansing and debridement, closed reduction if possible or open reduction with fixation, splinting with resin, and temporary filling with $Ca(OH)_2$—calcium hydroxyapatite—until the tissues have healed. A root canal treatment, definitive filling with gutta percha, or tooth restoration may be carried out after about 6 months. Poor dental or oral hygiene, medical comorbidities, severe injuries, poor general condition, and time elapsed between injury and treatment are significant factors in the survival of the affected teeth. Usually tooth elements do not survive beyond 2 h in the absence of active management. Saline, saliva, milk, or Hank's solution may be used to temporarily preserve teeth injured in trauma until definitive treatment can be carried out. In case of doubt, it is better to sacrifice the severely damaged tooth in risk of necrosis than to attempt replantation. Dentures may be advised after complete remodeling of the alveolar bone in approximately 6 months.

5.2.15 Face Transplant

Severe trauma to the face is a life-changing condition and that is an understatement. Along with considerable impairment of speech and articulation, it snatches away the identity of the individual, and in most instances, the quality of the life gained is worse than that which has been lost forever. It is practically impossible to live with the unimaginable disfigurement of the face and virtually mortifying to put up with endless rounds of multiple surgeries to restore an acceptable appearance.

Facial transplantation has partially solved this problem with the concept of face "replacement" as opposed to facial "restoration", but serious ethical problems come in the way of wide application of this method across the globe [27]. Facial transplantation is based on the concept of the angioneurosome or the specific patterns of blood and nerve supply to the facial architecture. It allows the facial skin cover to be harvested for use in another individual and thus minimize the need for multiple and staged surgeries.

In the medical and scientific sense, the single-stage nature of this surgical option offers considerable benefits over staged surgeries, and facial transplantation is being increasingly scrutinized and practiced in regions where the ethical issues have been handled to a large extent [28].

The ethical aspects of this procedure not only pertain to the recipient of the transplant but also the donor, the friends and family of both, and the wider society. The psychosocial parameters are therefore extremely important to consider and assess prior to undertaking this momentous decision [29].

The face transplant may be aided by adjunctive surgical procedures such as microvascular free flaps and the use of osseointegrated implants [30, 31]. This is especially useful in partial reconstruction or failure of the primary procedure due to rejection or graft-versus-host disease (GVHD).

5.3   Best Practice Recommendations

- In recent times the use of the subciliary approach to access the orbit is continually decreasing, as the transconjunctival route is gaining popularity because it provides a better cosmetic appearance [32]. Thus the first and foremost consideration in the treatment of trauma to the face is the optimal restoration of form (appearance) followed closely by function.
- Repair with an autologous graft provides a smooth and seamless integration and a low rate of extrusion, but the time taken for surgery is longer and the donor site morbidity is considerable [33].
- Many types of alloplastic implants are available, including absorbable and nonresorbable materials [34]. The primary repair should be done within 3–6 months after the acute injury so as to optimize restoration of facial appearance [35]. Calcium hydroxyapatite is available in injectable form, and dermal fillers, hyaluronic acid, and hydrophilic hydrogel pellets may be used as tissue self-expanders.
- In children utmost care must be taken while fixing plates and screws for the treatment of fractures so as not to harm the primary dentition. Maxilla-mandibular fixation (MMF) and open reduction with internal fixation (ORIF) may be required for orthognathic surgery, and various degrees of orthodontic correction may also be required for the treatment of malocclusion arising from trauma.
- Dentoalveolar injuries are often missed or not adequately treated in time even though they constitute an important aspect of facial trauma and are also quite common [36, 37]. They are very often encountered in cases of child abuse and thus should be looked into with special care and attention [38]. Many a time, they are seen in closed traumatic brain injuries, especially in children, and the consequences upon the primary dentition may be serious [39]. In older children with permanent dentition, enamel cracks may persist as a result of the previously suffered acute trauma [40].

Conclusion

Nasal and facial trauma is complex not only because of the peculiar structural anatomy but also the different types of tissues involved, all of which play crucial roles in trauma.

References

1. Evans BG, Evans GR. MOC-PSSM CME article: Zygomatic fractures. Plast Reconstr Surg. 2008;121(Suppl 1):1–11.
2. Fraioli RE, Branstetter BF, Deleyiannis FW. Facial fractures: beyond Le Fort. Otolaryngol Clin N Am. 2008;41(1):51–76.
3. Sweet CA. A classification and treatment for traumatized anterior teeth. ASDC J Dent Child. 1955;22:144–9.
4. Jain L, Qureshi S, Maurya A, et al. Hand dominance and blood group: association in epistaxis. Indian J Otolaryngol Head Neck Surg. 2017;69:121.
5. Ziu M, Savage JG, Jimenez DF. Diagnosis and treatment of cerebrospinal fluid rhinorrhoea following accidental traumatic skull base fractures. Neurosurg Focus. 2012;32(6):E3.
6. Sakas DE, Beale DJ, Ameen AA, Whitwell HL, Whittaker KW, Krebs AJ, et al. Compound anterior cranial base fractures: classification using computerized tomography scanning as a basis for selection of patients for dural repair. J Neurosurg. 1998;88:471–7.
7. van den Bergh B, Goey Y, Forouzanfar T. Postoperative radiographs after maxillofacial trauma: sense or nonsense? Int J Oral Maxillofac Surg. 2011;40:1373–6.
8. Ibrahim AM, Rabie AN, Lee BT, Lin SJ. Intraoperative CT: a teaching tool for the management of complex facial fracture fixation in surgical training. J Surg Educ. 2011;68:437–41.
9. Eljamel MS, Pidgeon CN. Localization of inactive cerebrospinal fluid fistulas. J Neurosurg. 1995;83:795–8.
10. Poduval J, Arokiaraj MC, Bhat V, Savery N. Bilateral sphenopalatine embolization in Panfacial fractures- a case report. Int J Coll Res Int Med Pub Heal (IJCRIMPH). 2013;5(1):30–6.
11. Rodriguez ED, Stanwix MG, Nam AJ, St Hilaire H, Simmons OP, Christy MR, et al. Twenty-six-year experience treating frontal sinus fractures: a novel algorithm based on anatomical fracture pattern and failure of conventional techniques. Plast Reconstr Surg. 2008;22(6):1850–66.
12. Smith TL, Han JK, Loehrl TA, Rhee JS. Endoscopic management of the frontal recess in frontal sinus fractures: a shift in the paradigm? Laryngoscope. 2002;112(5):784–90.
13. Schlosser RJ, Bolger WE. Nasal cerebrospinal fluid leaks: critical review and surgical considerations. Laryngoscope. 2004;114:255–65.
14. Kirtane MV, Gautham K, Upadhyaya SR. Endoscopic CSF rhinorrhoea closure: our experience in 267 cases. Otolaryngol Head Neck Surg. 2005;132:208–12.
15. Kim E, Russell PT. Prevention and management of skull base injury. Otolaryngol Clin N Am. 2010;43:809–16.
16. Castro B, Walcott BP, Redjal N, Coumans JV, Nahed BV. Cerebrospinal fluid fistula prevention and treatment following frontal sinus fractures: a review of initial management and outcomes. Neurosurg Focus. 2012;32(6):4.
17. Dhepnorrarat RC, Subramaniam S, Sethi DS. Endoscopic surgery for fronto-ethmoidal mucoceles: a 15-year experience. Otolaryngol Head Neck Surg. 2012;147(2):345–50.
18. Al-Qudah M, Graham SM. Modified osteoplastic flap approach for frontal sinus disease. Ann Otol Rhinol Laryngol. 2012;121(3):192–6.
19. Wallis A, Donald PJ. Frontal sinus fractures: a review of 72 cases. Laryngoscope. 1988;98:593–8.

20. Perry M. Maxillofacial trauma- developments, innovations and controversies. Injury. 2008;40(12):1252–9.
21. Meslemani D, Kellman RM. Zygomatico maxillary complex fractures. Arch Facial Plast Surg. 2012;14(1):62–6.
22. Ellis E, Throckmorton GS. Treatment of mandibular condylar process fractures: biological considerations. J Oral Maxillofac Surg. 2005;63:115–34.
23. Ellis E, Kellman RM, Vural E. Subcondylar fractures. Facial Plast Surg Clin North Am. 2012;20:365–82.
24. Ducic Y. Endoscopic treatment of subcondylar fractures. Laryngoscope. 2008;118:1164–7.
25. Goth S, Sawatari Y, Peleg M. Management of pediatric mandible fractures. J Craniofac Surg. 2012;23(1):47–56.
26. Siy RW, Brown RH, Koshy JC, et al. General management considerations in pediatric facial fractures. J Craniofac Surg. 2011;22(4):1190–5.
27. Alexander AJ, Alam DS, Gullane PJ, Lenqele BG, Adamson PA. Arguing the ethics of facial transplantation. Arch Facial Plast Surg. 2010;12(1):60–3.
28. Lantieri L, Hivelin M, Audard V, Benjoar MD, Meningaud JP, Bellivier F, Ortonne N, Lefaucheur JP, Gilton A, Suberbielle C, Marty J, Lang P, Grimbert P. Feasibility, reproducibility, risks and benefits of face transplantation: a prospective study of outcomes. Am J Transplant. 2011;11:367–78.
29. Soni CV, Barker JH, Pushpakumar SB, et al. Psychosocial considerations in facial transplantation. Burns. 2010;36:959–64.
30. Shipchandler TZ, Waters HH, Knott PD, Fritz MA. Orbitomaxillary reconstruction using the layered fibular osteo-cutaneous flap. Arch Facial Plast Surg. 2012;14(2):110–5.
31. Urken ML, Buchbinder D, Weinberg H, Vickery C, Sheiner A, Biller HF. Primary placement of osseointegrated implants in microvascular mandibular reconstruction. Otolaryngol Head Neck Surg. 1989;101:56.
32. Gosau M, Schoneich M, Draenert FG, Ettl T, Driemel O, Reichert TE. Retrospective analysis of orbital floor fractures- complications, outcome and review of literature. Clin Oral Investig. 2011;15(3):305–13.
33. Goiato MC, Demathe A, Suzuki T, dos Santos DM, de Carvalho Dekon SF. Management of orbital reconstruction. J Craniofac Surg. 2010;21:1834–6.
34. Gierloff M, Seeck GK, Springer I, Becker S, Kandzia C, Wiltfang J. Orbital floor reconstruction with resorbable polydioxanone implants. J Craniofac Surg. 2012;23:161–4.
35. Imola MJ, Ducic Y, Adelson RT. The secondary correction of post-traumatic craniofacial deformities. Otolaryngol Head Neck Surg. 2008;139:654–60.
36. Glendor U. Epidemiology of traumatic dental injuries- a 12 year review of the literature. Dent Traumatol. 2008;24(6):603–11.
37. Laskin DM. The recognition of child abuse. J Oral Surg. 1978;36:349.
38. Davidoff G, Jakubowski M, Thomas D, Alpert M. The spectrum of closed-head injuries in facial trauma victims: incidence and impact. Ann Emerg Med. 1988;17:27.
39. Ravn JJ. Sequelae of acute mechanical trauma in the primary dentition. J Dent Child. 1968;35(4):281–9.
40. Ravn JJ. Follow-up study of permanent incisors with enamel cracks as a result of acute trauma. Scand J Dent Res. 1981;89(2):117–23.

Trauma to the Neck and Aerodigestive Tract

Learning Objectives
- To learn the pathophysiology of trauma to the neck and aerodigestive tract
- To understand the clinical implications of management of trauma to the neck
- To remember the best practice recommendations in neck and aerodigestive trauma

6.1 Pathophysiology

6.1.1 Relevant Anatomy and Epidemiology

The larynx is a semirigid tubular structure in the neck that acts as a conduit for breathing, voicing, and swallowing, but the principal function of the larynx is to act as a protective sphincter for the lower airway and prevent aspiration into the lungs. It is about 44 mm in length, 43 mm in breadth, and 36 mm in the antero-posterior direction or sagittal plane in the male and 36, 41, and 26 mm in the same dimensions respectively, in the female. In infants and children, the subglottic portion of the larynx is the narrowest both structurally and because of mucosal laxity, while the glottis portion or the space between the vocal cords is the narrowest dimension in adults. The thyroid cartilages of both the sides join in the midline at an angle of 90° in the male and 120° in the female. This acute angulation in the male forms the Adam's apple and may be obscured or lost in the event of external trauma. The cricoid cartilage is signet shaped, being broader posteriorly than anteriorly, and is the only complete cartilaginous ring in the entire airway. This has serious implications in trauma because loss of or injury to the cricoid cartilage results in progressive and recalcitrant scarring and fibrosis which is virtually impossible to treat or may require multiple and difficult surgeries.

© Springer Nature Singapore Pte Ltd. 2018   117
J. Das, *Trauma in Otolaryngology*, https://doi.org/10.1007/978-981-10-6361-9_6

The thyroid and cricoid cartilages as well as the arytenoid cartilages (expect the apices) are composed of hyaline cartilage which starts to calcify in late adolescence and early adulthood. Thus areas of calcification in the upper airway, especially in the posterior aspects, may be mistaken for foreign bodies. Traumatic injuries to the external laryngeal nerve may result in a cord palsy on that side, with the affected vocal cord lying at a lower level than on the normal side and having a lax or wavy surface, due to the loss of tensioning by the cricothyroid muscle. Foreign bodies in the bronchi tend to impact more commonly on the right side, it being shorter, wider, and more in line with the trachea.

The incidence of trauma to the larynx is believed to range from 1 per 5000 to 15,000 depending on demographic factors. As may be expected, acute injuries to the larynx are seen more commonly in younger patients in case of environmental trauma but may span practically all age groups as far as iatrogenic airway trauma is concerned.

While it is somewhat comforting to know that penetrating trauma constitutes less than 5% of cases and blunt less than 1%, the outcomes of management of laryngeal trauma could be extremely poor if sound scientific principles are not kept in mind. This fact escapes most emergency care specialists, and it is probably in the effective treatment of airway injury that the expertise of otolaryngologists in general, and laryngologists and airway surgeons in particular, is especially required.

Below 40 years of age, when the thyroid cartilage is still unossified, the impact causes the larynx to be compressed against the cervical spine, splaying the thyroid cartilage. Upon relief of pressure, the elastic recoil of the thyroid cartilage causes it to split in the midline where the angulation is acute and the lines of force weak. This happens especially in males, as the female larynx is softer, more elastic, and more rounded in contour. Such a midline breach can avulse the epiglottis and vocal cords and even the arytenoid complexes. These structures may be contused, swollen, and hanging loose in the airway, causing dysphonia, pain and bleeding, and airway obstruction. As edema and inflammation develop over the next few hours following an injury, airway compromise may not occur at the outset and may be missed, especially when there are other life-threatening injuries requiring immediate attention. A high index of suspicion and continued vigilance alone would avoid such an unfortunate complication, especially as the patient is gradually settled into a stable position.

The larynx is usually well protected in the neck but is nevertheless vulnerable to trauma, especially motor vehicle or road traffic accidents. Seat belt and car safety regulations notwithstanding, such injuries are still quite common, especially in countries where such legislation is loosely enforced. Contact sports and personal assault are more common causes. As far as vehicular etiology is concerned, the larynx is more likely to be injured if the driver or passenger is tall, such that the neck is in direct line with the dashboard or steering wheel, and an acceleration-deceleration force throws the exposed neck and larynx hard onto the impacting surface.

Older adults whose larynges are partially ossified suffer similar injuries, with the additional features of flattening of the neck due to shattering of a rigid larynx and telescoping of its fragments. In either case, loss of neck contour is seen due to loss of the thyroid prominence, and surgical emphysema may be found if the airway lumen has been breached by mucosal injury.

Fracture of the hyoid may occur in cases of strangulation, throttling, and garroting and less commonly in hanging. The hyoid may be extremely tender and have a "springing" effect on palpation, though such an injury does not require anything more than a conservative approach if occurring in isolation.

The presence of a ligature line and other soft tissue injuries over the neck must be looked for. Subcutaneous emphysema may be present in a hyoid fracture, and crepitus due to the fragments of bone may be evident. Mucosal edema and/or hematoma may be present, and one must be vigilant for airway obstruction in such cases. Though the anatomy of the neck is somewhat distorted by hyoid fracture, it is not deemed an emergency and does not require repair in the form of either open or closed reduction and/or reconstruction, as the hyoid bone is not indispensable to breathing, swallowing, or voicing.

6.1.2 Laryngeal Trauma Can Be Classified into Five Grades

Laryngeal trauma can be classified into five grades based on the Schaefer-Fuhrman system:

1. *I—small hematoma* within the laryngeal mucosa, no obvious fracture.
2. *II—hematoma, edema, and small breaks* in the mucosa but no cartilage exposed, fracture noted on CT scan but no displacement seen.
3. *III—widespread and severe edema,* tears in the mucosa, exposure of cartilage, and immobility (paralysis or fixation) of cord.
4. *IV—above, with more than two sites* in the larynx involved, severe lacerations of mucosa.
5. *V—total separation* of the larynx from the trachea.

Laryngotracheal trauma may thus range from edema and hematoma to tears, lacerations, fractures, vocal cord immobility, and complete separation from the lower airway. Grade 1 is minor trauma without exposure of cartilage and fractures. Grade 2 is more severe trauma with edema and hematoma with non-displaced fractures but without cartilage exposure. Grade 3 is severe trauma with displaced fracture(s), cartilage exposure, and/or vocal cord immobility. Grade 4 is even more severe trauma with unstable fractures immediately threatening the airway, and grade 5 is laryngotracheal separation which is potentially fatal.

While the classification of the severity of laryngotracheal injury is given above, the various modalities of neck and airway injury include:

1. Cut-throat attacks
2. Clothesline injuries
3. Throttling and strangulation
4. Hanging—partial and complete

5. Whiplash and cervical spine injury
6. Inhalation injury
7. Iatrogenic—airway instrumentation
8. Ballistic wounds
9. Miscellaneous—surgical scars, insect bites, and foreign bodies
10. Phonotrauma

The neck has been divided into three zones as far as trauma is concerned, but zone 2 can be considered to be the neck proper, that is, the region between the mandible and cricoid. This zone is normally prevented from trauma by virtue of automatic flexion of the neck in most modes of injury so that the bony prominences of the facial skeleton and chest wall bear the brunt of the insult. But there are many other modes of injury where the neck is directly exposed and which cause penetrating or blunt airway trauma.

6.1.3 The Neck May Be Divided into Three Zones

The neck may be divided into three zones for the purpose of simplifying the process of management:

1. *Below the cricoid cartilage* (lower neck)—the contents are the carotid, vertebral and subclavian arteries, lung, trachea and esophagus, thoracic duct, and mediastinal contents.
2. *In between the cricoid and mandible* (midneck)—the contents are the carotid and vertebral arteries, jugular veins, larynx, trachea and esophagus, recurrent laryngeal, ansa cervicalis, and vagus nerves.
3. *Above the mandible* (upper neck)—the contents are the carotid (distal portion) and vertebral arteries, jugular veins, parotid and submandibular glands, and last four cranial nerves (9–12).

Zone 2 is different from the other two because it is principally composed of soft tissue with the vertebral column posteriorly being the only bony component. The laryngeal skeleton in front offers some structural rigidity to the neck but not protection. The muscles of the neck however are distributed in an overlapping and circular fashion, and the natural tendency is to flex the neck in the event of an external insult. This mechanism offers some degree of protection to the neck but is not adequate in the face of many types of trauma, especially penetrating injury as seen in cut-throat (stab wounds), gunshot wounds, or lacerated wounds with shrapnel or flying debris and blunt trauma due to motor vehicle accidents (MVA), strangulation, or sports injuries, external injuries from chemical or thermal burns, and last but not the least inhalation injuries with steam and gases.

Zone 3 injuries mainly involve the lower jaw and deeper aspects of the facial skeleton and have been described separately. Zone 1 trauma is the commonest type, most likely to be seen in cases of polytrauma, and may thus also involve significant trauma to the chest wall, thorax, and mediastinum, and is therefore beyond the purview of the otolaryngologist alone, and would involve thoracic and general surgeons for its management.

Injuries in zones 1 and 3 are relatively more common than in zone 2 but are more difficult to treat as access is restricted by elements of the bony skeleton in these areas. Zone 2, even though naturally protected, is exposed substantially in many situations, and this carries serious implications because of the presence of the airway and upper aerodigestive tract and important vascular and neural structures. Trauma to these structures can be life-threatening, but if detected and treated promptly, it carries a good prognosis. Surgical access, exposure, and control of the injured area(s) are much easier than in the other two zones.

The important structures lying in zone 3 and potentially at risk in neck trauma are the major vessels of the neck such as the internal carotid artery (ICA), external carotid artery (ECA), internal jugular vein (IJV), external jugular vein (EJV), the anterior jugular veins, nerves such as the lower four cranial nerves and the ansa hypoglossi, and the superior limit of the brachial plexus, the larynx and trachea, the thyroid gland, and the pharynx and esophagus. Injuries to the spine and vertebral column are not discussed here. The muscles of the neck may be involved along with damage to the other structures mentioned above.

6.1.4 Injury to the Salivary Glands

Injury to the salivary glands may be seen in zone 3 injuries to the neck. Unfortunately, most of these injuries may be missed during the acute assessment and control of trauma, in favor of more serious injuries. Thus trauma to the salivary glands is usually manifested as a late sequel or complication. Other causes of injury to the salivary glands, such as that arising from surgery or radiation therapy, are more readily detected or anticipated, and timely action can be taken in these cases.

The major salivary glands—parotid, submandibular, and sublingual—may be injured in penetrating trauma, whereby injury to the gland, duct, or nerve supply may occur. Injury to the gland results in a salivary leak, that to the duct results in a stricture with formation of a sialocele, and that to the nerve supply causes problems of dryness and difficulty in mastication, which lead further to the complications of xerostomia such as gingivitis and periodontitis.

Injury to minor salivary glands may coexist along with major salivary gland trauma or be seen as an isolated incident in case of cheek and mucosal bites or plugging of the duct opening with epithelial debris. The latter could be due to alterations in the mucosa of the upper aerodigestive tract due to various external stimuli such as foodstuffs, smoking, alcohol abuse, reflux esophagitis or gastroesophageal reflux, systemic diseases such as scleroderma or other collagen disorders, and the effect of medications or radiation treatments. Minor salivary gland trauma can cause retention cysts and resultant discomfort and a foreign body sensation or "feeling of something in the throat" (FOSIT). Surgical removal is required if the cyst is large and/or symptomatic and also as prophylaxis against the potential development of carcinoma resulting from chronic irritation.

A salivary leak may be missed in acute trauma as the saliva is likely to be admixed with blood. If obvious damage to the gland, duct, or nerve is detected, then the presence of saliva may be confirmed with an estimation of the amylase levels in the blood or secretions. Plain X-rays may help to detect debris such as pieces of shrapnel; foreign bodies such as wood, metal, and glass; impacted teeth or bone; and so on. Computerized tomography (CT) scan is the method of choice for the detection of bone and soft tissue injuries in the surrounding area, but a more detailed search for injury to the gland, duct, or nerve would be better with the help of magnetic resonance imaging (MRI).

6.1.5   Blunt Laryngeal Trauma

The etiology and epidemiology include direct physical assault (punching, throttling, strangling, contact sports), accidental trauma (clothesline injuries, traffic injuries as seen in motorbike riders driving at high speed and suffering an impact against a fixed obstacle such as barricade), suicidal injuries (hanging), and the deceleration type of injury with the neck extended so that the larynx is exposed and vulnerable (such as that occurring in whiplash injuries).

Hard impact causes the stiff laryngeal skeleton to shatter, resulting in a comminuted fracture. Movement of the fracture fragments and direct transmission of force to the deeper tissues cause mucosal avulsion and tears of the mucosa of the upper aerodigestive tract.

Communication between the air-filled cavities and potential spaces of the neck causes subcutaneous emphysema which can track even into the deep neck spaces of the retropharyngeal compartment and superior mediastinum and can prove fatal (Fig. 6.1).

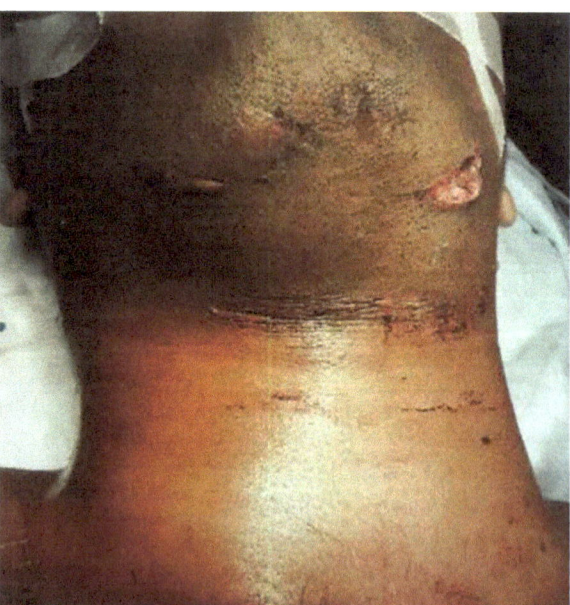

Fig. 6.1 Subcutaneous emphysema obscuring neck landmarks

Throttling and strangulation are usually homicidal in nature, and the soft tissues of the neck and cartilages of the larynx are subjected to blunt forces resulting in considerable amounts of contusion, and even fractures of the hyoid, thyroid, and cricoid may occur. Bleeding into the lumen of the airway and mucosal hematomas are common and result in fatality by respiratory obstruction and hypoxia.

Hanging may be suicidal, homicidal, or accidental and occur by either partial or complete modes. Partial hanging occurs when the feet are in contact with the ground or any other surface thus resulting in incomplete suspension and therefore milder degrees of injury. Complete hanging refers to total suspension of the body in air allowing it to hang by gravity and is invariably fatal as it results in atlanto-axial dislocation and depression of the respiratory center in the medulla. However, the effects of hanging start setting in at the very early stages itself when the neck undergoes compression. Arterial supply is thus interrupted resulting in hypoxia, followed by venous congestion which can cause capillary hemorrhages and exacerbate the hypoxia and acidosis. Respiratory depression and a fall in the sensorium occur, resulting in unconsciousness. If the victim is not rescued in time, the situation deteriorates further ultimately leading to coma and death. The ligature mark is usually above the level of the hyoid bone thus sparing it and all the other structures of the neck.

Though cricoarytenoid joint subluxation or dislocation has usually been described in the background of intubation trauma, it may also be seen in blunt external neck trauma in the rare instance [1].

6.1.6 Penetrating Laryngeal Trauma

Cut-throat injuries of the neck may occur due to suicidal, homicidal, or accidental events and range from superficial to deep and thus involve various structures. All, however, typically tend to be serious, even fatal. A superficial slash across the neck may bleed for a short time if the injury is only skin deep. In this case, the skin and the underlying platysma are usually cut together, and no major vessels are involved. If the wound is irregular, subcutaneous emphysema may occur due to air trapping, leading to a substantial compression of the soft tissues of the neck and consequently respiratory obstruction. Deeper wounds typically bleed for longer times as major arteries and veins are involved and thus quickly cause exsanguination, leading to hemodynamic collapse, shock, and unconsciousness due to brain hypoxia. Blood and salivary secretions can enter or pool in the airway and result in respiratory compromise, but this might be amenable to endotracheal intubation if facilities for suction are available.

Clothesline injuries are similar to cut-throat attacks except that the wound may be more clearly defined. At the same time, soft tissue contusion may be significant depending on proximity, velocity, and gravity. Motorcycle riders and bicyclists are most at risk of clothesline injuries, and in domestic settings the inciting agent (clothesline) is relatively at close range, hitting the victim at moderate velocity, and is usually free from additional factors such as glass pieces. On the other hand, in many countries where kite flying is a recreational and cultural sport, pieces of glass or tile may be stuck to the kite string to weigh it down and give it tension and facilitate kite floatation. Practitioners or spectators of such sport may be victims of the clothesline type of injuries as they look up to the skies and track the kite(s), thus exposing the neck when the kite comes swooping down. Such injuries must be treated along the same lines as other cut-throats, except that mass casualties are common.

Penetrating trauma to the neck is more amenable to timely treatment as the injury and its impact are self-evident. In the case of blunt trauma, much of the injury may be deep or hidden and may elude early diagnosis, particularly in the background of other injuries. However, the consequences of missing such injuries are enormous. Apart from an unstable airway, complications arising from esophageal injury may claim the patient's life even after all other injuries have been taken care of.

The type of neck trauma usually varies from setting to setting. Penetrating injuries are common in outdoor scenarios and commonly associated with sociodemographic factors, closely followed by blunt neck trauma [2, 3]. Tracheotomy is the preferred procedure prior to commencement of definitive treatment for the injury. Complications such as wound infection, fistula formation, and scarring or stenosis are rather common in this kind of trauma if the primary repair has been suboptimal. Close follow-up with endoscopy is essential for the prompt detection and treatment of complications.

6.1.7 The Presenting Signs and Symptoms of Neck Injury

The presenting signs and symptoms of neck injury have been divided into soft and hard signs widely known as the Rosen criteria, as a guide to planning optimal management of the patient.

The soft signs are:

1. Blood-stained oral secretions
2. Hemoptysis and/or hematemesis
3. Stridor or dyspnea or respiratory distress
4. Change in voice (dysphonia) or difficulty in swallowing (dysphagia)
5. Subcutaneous or surgical emphysema in the neck (crepitations)
6. Soft tissue contusion/bruising/or a stable hematoma in the neck
7. Focal neurological deficit(s)
8. Air in the mediastinum (airway injury) or chest wall (leaking intercostal or chest tube)—as seen on imaging

The hard signs are:

1. Acute airway obstruction
2. Active and significant bleeding
3. Hypovolemic shock resistant to fluid replacement
4. Rapidly expanding neck hematoma

5. Radial pulse feeble or absent
6. Vascular thrill (on palpation) or bruit (on auscultation) in the neck
7. Evidence of brain hypoxia or ischemia

In any kind of neck trauma, it is important to keep in mind the involvement of vascular and neural structures passing through the neck, the anterior compartment comprising of the airway, and the posterior compartment consisting of the vertebral column. This is an arbitrary division but helps to decide which elements are involved and which specialty should be called in first to deal with the situation.

Thus if there is marked bleeding from a neck wound, a cardiothoracic vascular consult would be needed urgently. Similarly, the presence of quadriparesis or quadriplegia warrants a neurosurgical or orthopedic opinion primarily. Needless to say, the ENT surgeon is almost always involved in the primary assessment in order to determine the status of the airway and so is the anesthetist in most cases.

Open neck exploration may prove challenging when concomitant injury to the cervical spine has also occurred. In these cases, a cervical collar which might have been put in place to stabilize the spine may interfere with surgical access and exposure of the neck. In accordance with the NEXUS (National Emergency X-Radiography Utilization Study) criteria, the cervical collar may be removed in a negative neck, that is, when the following are present:

1. No midline spine tenderness
2. No focal neurological deficit
3. No painful distracting injury
4. No intoxication
5. Normal alertness

These criteria are by and large applicable to most situations but may be less reliable in elderly patients (above the age of 65 years). The Canadian C-spine Rule may be used as an alternative for decision making. CT imaging would be the final yardstick for determining the extent of trauma to the cervical spine and should be employed whenever feasible. Close monitoring with neurosurgery consult and maintaining the cervical collar, at the same time avoiding oral feeding and maintaining the patient in the intensive care unit (ICU), are advisable.

6.1.8 Inhalation Trauma

Airway trauma can also occur as a result of inhalation of hot air, steam, liquids, and noxious substances. Various patterns of inhalation injury may be seen depending on the nature of the injurious agent. While hot air or gas tends to affect the supraglottic areas first as this is the first region of the larynx to come in contact with the inhalant, hot air rich in humidity, such as steam, affects the subglottic area, trachea, bronchi, and bronchioles as it tends to travel further down the airway. Smoke, however, tends to affect the entire respiratory tract by causing chemical injury. It results in loss of surfactant and produces ARDS (acute respiratory distress syndrome)-like symptoms and signs. Inhalation trauma may occur in isolation but is more commonly seen in complex injuries including industrial injuries and motor vehicle accidents. A less obvious but perhaps more ominous inhalation injury is caused by smoking, both active and passive.

6.1.9 Iatrogenic Trauma

Iatrogenic trauma is the term given to the entity where trauma occurs due to medical intervention or medical error, and in the case of the larynx, it is fast emerging as a major cause of trauma [4]. This is very simple to understand if one recalls that in the modern era of medical care, long-term endotracheal intubation is almost a given in most situations—be it in the management of trauma or other illnesses—and this constitutes one of the biggest instances of airway injury.

This is due to the unique anatomical structure and physiological function of the larynx. Most of the laryngeal skeleton is elastic and expandable because of the cartilage and muscular components, except in the region of the cricoid ring, which is the only complete cartilaginous ring in the entire larynx. The cartilage has extremely poor ability to heal and regenerate, and when it does, it is always with the formation of fibrous or scar tissue. The cartilage therefore must be prevented from injury and exposure by taking utmost care in order to preserve the mucosa of the larynx and trachea.

At a pressure of 30 mm Hg, the microcirculation of laryngeal mucosa is cut off, and it suffers necrosis, exposing the cartilage underneath. There is an inflammatory reaction in the cartilage, or perichondritis, leading to the formation of granulation tissue which eventually organizes into a circumferential scar. In fact, scar tissue formation is rather florid and relentless in the larynx, much like a hypertrophic scar on the skin surface. It is only a subtle balance between regeneration and fibrosis that would maintain the integrity of the airway, and this process is highly unpredictable. Thus every attempt must be made to ensure that the viability of the laryngeal mucosa is preserved to the maximum extent possible.

The mechanisms of iatrogenic laryngeal trauma are different from external laryngeal injury, which may be blunt, penetrating, or due to inhalation of toxic substances. The diagnosis depends on the acute symptoms and direct and indirect signs and mandates the securing of the airway first and foremost. The principles of basic life support (BLS) and advanced trauma life support (ATLS) must be followed religiously. Diagnosis is greatly aided by flexible fiber optic laryngoscopy (FFL) and imaging by computerized tomography (CT) scan.

Endotracheal intubation is a ubiquitous procedure in all emergency and critical care settings and has indeed been revolutionary in saving lives. However, it is not without its perils, and iatrogenic airway trauma due to intubation and tracheotomy is increasingly on the rise. The factors influencing trauma due to intubation are its duration, the size of the tube used, the pressure in the cuff, friction between the tube and the airway mucosa due to movements caused by patient agitation or a short connector between the patient and the ventilator, repeated attempts at intubation, foreign body reaction due to the material used in the tube, release of toxic substances from the tube especially during autoclaving or sterilization of the tubes that are used multiple times in the same or different patients, the use of a stylet during intubation, route of intubation whether oral or nasotracheal, the nursing care given, and, last but not least, demographic factors such as gender and age differences.

Even routine and seemingly minor endoscopic procedures have the potential to cause trauma. Some of the reasons for iatrogenic trauma while performing endoscopy are rough or inept handling of the instrument as is expected when less experienced persons such as resident doctors or trainees and junior staff are performing the procedure especially in unsupervised settings, using an inappropriately sized or oversized instrument, taking more than the minimally required tissue for the purpose of biopsy, and excessive or inappropriate use of laser.

Trauma may be due to nasogastric tube insertion caused by rough and forceful insertion especially in uncooperative patients; foreign body reaction due to the material used in the tube; swallowing problems such as cricopharyngeal spasm or mechanical causes such as strictures and tumors; pressure necrosis of the nasal ala especially if an oversized tube has been inserted or if the septum is deviated causing the tube to fit too tightly; gastroesophageal reflux disease (GERD) and laryngopharyngeal reflux (LPR), which may predispose to or cause ulceration of the mucosa; exposure and inflammation of the cartilage leading to perichondritis; and eventually fibrosis and contracture. Several causes of trauma may exist simultaneously, thus compounding their effects and leading to persistent injury. Some of these factors may even be missed, for example, when treating trauma survivors in critical care and subjecting them to various degrees of aerodigestive interventions.

6.1.10 Vocal Cord Paralysis

Damage to the recurrent laryngeal nerve on one or both sides may occur as a result of blunt or penetrating neck trauma and also as a result of iatrogenic injury as seen in thyroid or neck surgery and intubation trauma. While cricoarytenoid joint subluxation or dislocation may be treated primarily if detected in time, established paralysis must be treated with a combination of techniques.

Generally, compensation by the mobile cord in case of unilateral paralysis is sufficient for most of the patient's needs unless he or she is a professional voice user. Adequate time must elapse for spontaneous return of function, and this may take up to 1 year and may even be erratic or incomplete. Temporary measures such as injection laryngoplasty may be undertaken, or laryngeal framework surgery types 1 and 2 may be performed for permanent return of function. Laryngeal reinnervation techniques are emerging as the treatment for vocal cord paralysis caused by trauma in addition to other causes.

6.1.11 Phonotrauma

An important aspect of laryngeal trauma includes phonotrauma or voice-related trauma. This is often not described in detail in texts on trauma but merits discussion in this book simply by virtue of being an eminently preventable cause of morbidity, as perhaps all kinds of trauma are, in a manner of speaking (no pun intended!).

Phonotrauma broadly includes three entities—vocal cord nodules, vocal cord cysts, and vocal cord polyps. It may, in a larger sense, also encompass other injurious forms of laryngeal disorders such as vocal cord granulomas, contact ulcers, sulcus vocalis, and dysphonia plicae ventricularis.

Vocal abuse is the wrong or faulty use of one's voice by factors which may lead to unnatural stress and strain on the vocal apparatus—actions such as loud or effortful talking, shouting, screaming for long periods of time, or even whispering in order to be heard when voice rest has been advised as a treatment measure! It is common in habitual screamers, teachers or public speakers not using audiovisual aids, young mothers with children to care for, or those who are hard of hearing and do not have the benefit of auditory feedback to help modulate the quality of their voice.

Vocal overuse may occur in those who need to speak for prolonged periods of time much beyond their normal capacity or requirements, even with the help of audiovisual aids, for example, when a professional voice user has to deliver a long series of lectures, concerts, discourses, et cetera.

Vocal misuse, on the other hand, is defined by the use of one's voice for a specific purpose that may not be in accordance with his or her fundamental frequency—by training the vocal apparatus accordingly, as opera singers might do—and is not usually associated with the occurrence of vocal nodules.

Vocal nodules involve the medial or superficial part of the superficial lamina propria (SLP—also known as Reinke's space) and are composed of fibrous or scar tissue caused by friction at the cord margins in the event of long-standing vocal abuse. Vocal cord nodules are generally bilateral, although one side or the other may be involved earlier, and are symmetrical swellings found on the true vocal cord margins at their vibratory edge and roughly at the junction of the anterior one third and posterior two thirds of the membranous part of the vocal cord. They are also called teacher's, screamer's, or singer's nodules, signifying vocal abuse or overuse as the etiological factor.

A *vocal cord cyst* is usually unilateral and is in reality an epithelial inclusion or retention cyst caused by obstruction of the duct of a minor salivary gland present in the mucosa. The obstruction may be triggered by friction or inflammation resulting from vocal abuse or may be idiopathic in nature. The cyst grows large enough to cause disturbances of voice quality and distortion of the mucosal wave as seen on videostroboscopy. It is a benign lesion and must be differentiated from a more sinister pathology such as malignancy using specialized methods of investigation such as contact endoscopy, autofluorescence, optical coherence tomography (OCT), and, in recent times, high-speed imaging and narrowband imaging (NBI).

A *vocal polyp* may be sessile or pedunculated and is caused by prolapse of SLP through a minute breach on the mucosal surface, brought about by a single act of severe voice strain or by chronic or habitual shouting. The usual cause is hemorrhage of a capillary or venule into the submucosa, so in the acute condition, it appears red in color, or a blood vessel may be seen clearly over it. As it grows in the background of unabated voice abuse and failure to take treatment, it causes voice disturbances such as hoarseness and breathiness or sometimes stridor and problems with respiration if it prolapses into the subglottic space.

6.2   Clinical Implications

Stridor, bleeding through the mouth, cough, dysphagia, and odynophagia are common presenting symptoms. Surgical emphysema, neck swelling, bleeding, and respiratory distress are common signs. The basic principles of ATLS apply to neck trauma. The airway and breathing must be secured first and foremost by either endotracheal intubation or tracheotomy. Direct orotracheal intubation with laryngoscopy should be tried first as this will help to assess the airway as well as secure it at the same time. With the passage of time and/or repeated attempts, control of the airway becomes more and more compromised and may prove fatal. Rapid sequence intubation (RSI) can be tried if a skilled anesthetist is present at the scene. Nasotracheal intubation is successful only in the most experienced hands, is often a matter of luck, and should be avoided unless facilities for an awake fiber optic intubation are at hand. Tracheotomy is often lifesaving in these situations and must be undertaken expediently when doubt exists as to the state of the airway or in a rapidly deteriorating patient. Bleeding and/or brain hypoxia as seen in strangulation or hanging predisposes to adult respiratory distress syndrome (ARDS) or pulmonary edema, further complicating the acute crisis.

6.2.1   The Surgical Airway

Treatment of any trauma in general requires a secure airway, and a tracheotomy may be done to surgically create an airway when all other measures are unsuccessful or not feasible. *Tracheotomy* is performed by the following techniques:

1. Open surgical technique
2. Cricothyroidotomy or mini-tracheotomy
3. Percutaneous dilatational tracheotomy

The creation of a surgical airway carries with it the potential for iatrogenic trauma, and all the above procedures bear this risk. However, the planned or elective open surgical technique is generally performed by trained surgeons, and thus more control over the procedure is possible. The second one must be performed in an emergency situation and converted as soon as possible into a definitive tracheotomy, and the outcome would vary accordingly. It is only the third option that is being increasingly performed by medical professionals trained in emergency care but not necessarily trauma surgery. Thus it has been mentioned here in some detail.

Percutaneous dilatational tracheotomy (PDT) is a procedure by which tracheotomy is performed by a minimal access technique. A small horizontal skin incision of about 1centimeter is made at a level between the first and second tracheal ring after infiltrating the skin with a local anesthetic solution. A mosquito artery forceps is then used to release the soft tissues and gently separate the strap muscles of the neck in the midline until the shiny white pretracheal fascia is just visualized. A syringe half filled with saline or local anesthetic solution such as 4% lignocaine is used to confirm the position of the trachea by withdrawing the piston, when air bubbles may be seen in the syringe. At the same time, a few drops of the topical anesthetic are instilled into the tracheal lumen to prevent reflex bronchospasm. A guide wire is then introduced into the airway, preferably under fiber optic bronchoscopic guidance. A canula is passed over the guide wire, and the latter removed through it keeping the canula in situ. Dilators of increasing size are then passed over the canula until the largest dilator appropriate for the patient and the tracheotomy tube to be used have been passed easily and smoothly. Alternatively, a single dilator of varying diameters across its length, such as the Ciaglia Blue Rhino dilator, may be passed in a single stroke. Finally the tracheotomy tube is loaded on the dilator and inserted into the airway by the railroad or Seldinger technique, and the dilator removed. The tracheotomy tube is secured using skin stay sutures and/or tapes around the neck, and the patient connected to the ventilator or allowed to breathe spontaneously.

PDT evolved as an option for bedside tracheotomy in critically ill or moribund patients as a safer alternative to open bedside tracheotomy and its attendant risks and complications. However, it is not without its own dangers and contraindications, which include the following:

1. Patients requiring emergency tracheotomy
2. Unfavorable neck anatomy—cases where neck extension is not possible (as in cervical spondylosis or cervical trauma with atlantoaxial dislocation or subluxation), tumors or a large goiter over the neck, and patients with obesity and a short neck
3. Bleeding disorders with platelets less than 50,000 per cubic millimeter of blood or an INR (international normalized ratio) of more than 1.5
4. Patients requiring a positive end-expiratory pressure (PEEP) of more than 20 cm H_2O pressure

The PDT kit is also rather costly and the procedure more time-consuming than a standard open surgical tracheotomy. Therefore, it is only cost-effective in selected cases. The advantage is that emergency care physicians and those without a surgical background and training are able to perform this procedure safely and effectively.

The risk of subcutaneous emphysema is higher in PDT compared to an open procedure because the pretracheal fascia is not freed and incised and the trachea skeletonized as in open surgical tracheotomy, so strict vigilance must be maintained in the post procedure period, especially if the patient is on a ventilator. Comminuted fractures of the trachea are also quite common, and with such injuries, the risk of tracheal stenosis is abnormally high.

The size of Portex tube denotes its inner diameter, and the size of the suction catheter should not exceed more than half of the size of the tracheotomy tube. Tube placement must be confirmed by chest auscultation to see if air entry is bilaterally symmetrical unless it was abnormal at the outset. Doing a check X-ray after routine tracheotomy (open or PDT) is not borne out by evidence.

Cuff pressure must be maintained at 20–25 cm H_2O pressure, and care taken not to exceed 30 mm Hg or 30 cm water pressure, at which point the microcirculation in the laryngeal mucosa is known to cease. Accordingly, it is advisable to use intubation and tracheotomy tubes which have a low-pressure, high-volume cuff, as are commonly found nowadays, as against the earlier generation of tubes with low-volume, high-pressure cuffs. Morbidity associated with iatrogenic trauma, as may be seen in the case of tracheotomy, can be reduced with the adoption of techniques such as the minimally invasive tracheotomy [5].

Also, it is advisable to use the minimum size possible for ventilation instead of a large caliber tube, in order to minimize airway injury. Even then, airway instrumentation with techniques such as tracheotomy carries fatal risks such as tracheoesophageal fistula especially during the acute management of complicated trauma, and lesser forms of morbidity such as tracheo-cutaneous fistula in the healing phases (Fig. 6.2).

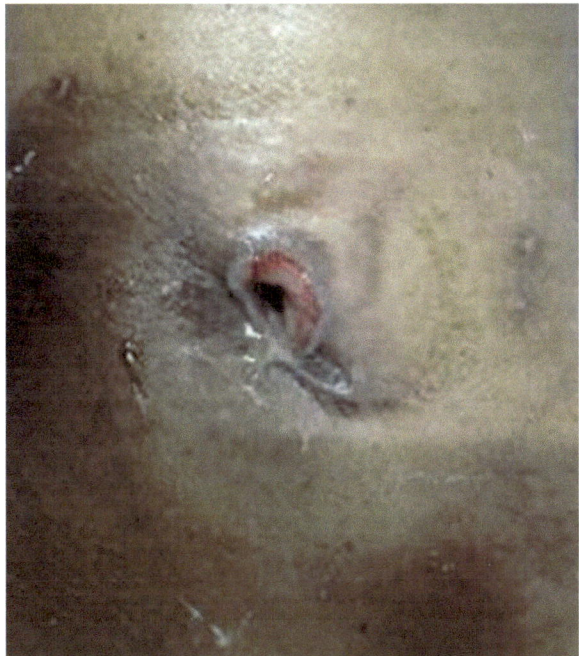

Fig. 6.2 Tracheo-cutaneous fistula

Only after the airway is under control is attention turned to bleeding and other issues, although swift and sometimes simultaneous control of both airway and bleeding are of the essence in a successful salvage. Tamponade or direct pressure over a bleeding vessel is a better idea than applying a clamp blindly over the affected area and causing collateral damage. The Trendelenburg position helps to avoid air embolism through an injured internal jugular vein but may worsen arterial bleeding, so careful judgment is necessary during patient positioning. Clots are best left undisturbed unless an open surgical exploration is already underway.

6.2.2   Treatment of Neck Trauma

Treatment of neck trauma also depends greatly on the symptoms and presentation. For example, severe hemorrhage from a neck wound, rapid swelling of the neck, stridor or obvious respiratory distress, neurological deficit, or altered sensorium call for management in a hospital at the earliest possible with the utmost care taken to transfer the patient without aggravating the situation further.

Clinical examination and plain radiographs may just show the tip of the iceberg, and CT scan of the neck, preferably with contrast if not otherwise contraindicated, would have to be done in the majority of cases of suspected laryngeal injury, followed by direct laryngoscopy and open neck exploration if necessary.

The diagnosis and management depend on a quick but methodical assessment of the injury. The primary survey will reveal the diagnosis, and immediate intervention must be done to secure the airway. Though a tracheotomy is desirable, it may be technically difficult to perform as an emergency measure. A cricothyrotomy is another option, but modern methods of intubation and the devices available make endotracheal intubation an equally safe choice if the persons performing the same have some degree of experience and are prepared for a difficult intubation owing to edema, bleeding and secretions, and a distorted anatomy. Intubation has the added advantage of providing an endoluminal stent and preventing further collapse and distortion of the airway.

Airway protection is mandatory, but care must be exercised to stabilize a cervical spine fracture if any by the use of a cervical collar with or without traction and avoidance of neck extension.

Similarly, passing a nasogastric is a hazardous prospect in these cases, but if accomplished successfully, it can stent and secure the digestive tract, seal small tears of the mucosa, and prevent reflux of potentially contaminating gastric contents into the site of trauma. Once the airway is secure, the secondary survey must meticulously assess the true extent of the injury and the presence of other injuries, if any.

Investigations include, apart from routine laboratory tests to assess the patient's nutritional and metabolic status, advance imaging procedures that need to be done to determine the exact nature and severity of the laryngeal trauma.

A CT scan with contrast is very useful. Virtual reality endobronchial simulation (VRES) or virtual bronchoscopy may be done where a direct visualization is not possible but this is less than ideal for the assessment of endoluminal injuries of subtle degrees. It is also a useful tool for further review and follow-up of the patient.

Plain and contrast high-resolution CT scan with bone windows will help to delineate fractures, the presence of air in the soft tissues suggesting mucosal lacerations, and soft tissue edema that narrows the airway lumen, as well as displacements, subluxations and dislocations of the joints and ligaments of the laryngeal skeleton, and injury to the cervical spine (Figs. 6.3, 6.4, 6.5).

CT angiography (CTA) using the 64-slice CT is considered the method of choice for imaging all the three neck zones as it is highly sensitive, is cost-effective in terms of cost and speed, and is convenient as it is relatively noninvasive compared to conventional angiography using the Seldinger technique. It may be employed in both penetrating and blunt trauma to the neck.

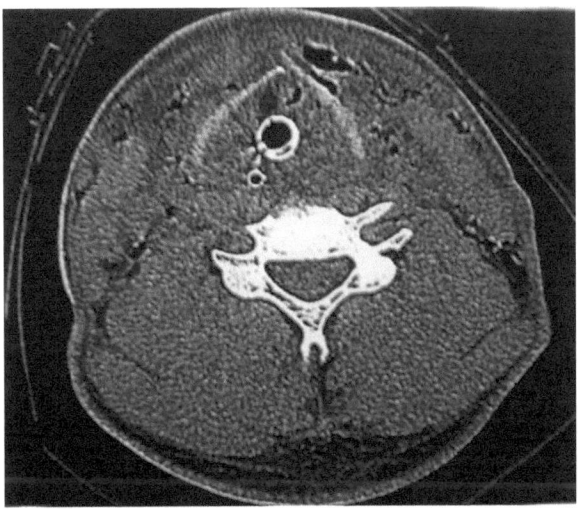

Fig. 6.3 Laryngeal fracture—axial view

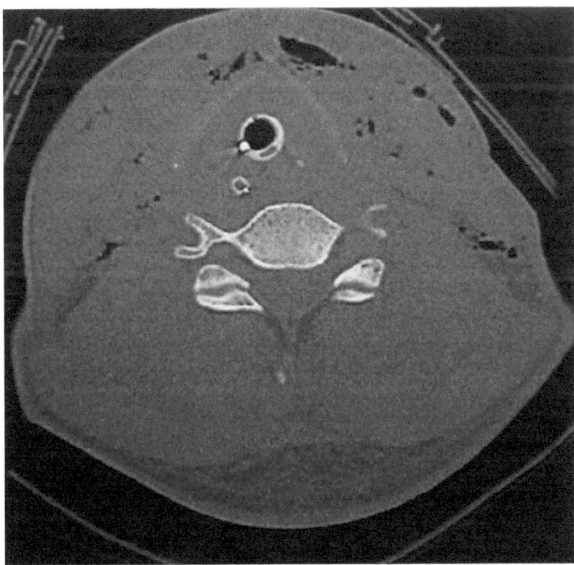

Fig. 6.4 Laryngeal fracture—bone window

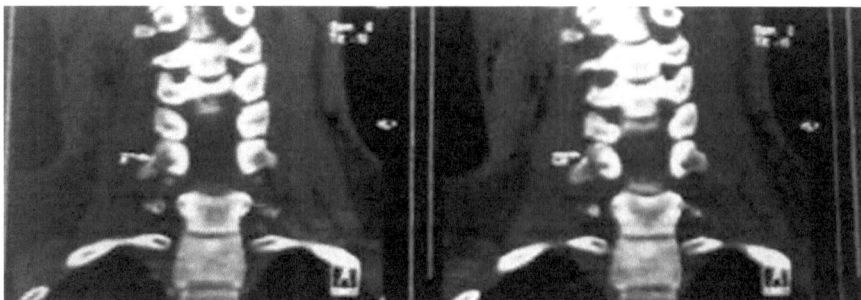

Fig. 6.5 Cervical spine fracture

Depending on the clinical and laryngoscopic findings and the results of imaging, appropriate management of the patient can be carried out. Grade I and II injuries may be treated conservatively with close observation toward sudden airway obstruction and with the help of antibiotics, proton pump inhibitors, corticosteroids, and inhalation of humidified air. The head end of the bed may be elevated to reduce congestion and prevent airway collapse as might be more common in the supine position. Heliox, which is a mixture of helium and oxygen in the ratio of 3:2, may make the effort of respiration lighter as helium lowers the specific gravity of the inspired air, but this is also known to mask impending airway obstruction and hence better avoided. Grade III injuries and above must be treated with open exploration and various procedures such as plating, wiring, stenting, and endoscopic repair. Plating with static or dynamic compression plates (DCP) such as miniplates and microplates is far superior to simply wiring the fracture fragments together, though the latter is a much simpler procedure to perform. This is because the fragments tend to move with respiration and swallowing and whenever the patient attempts to speak, and wires may either get loosened or displaced and the alignment thus disrupted. Plating also provides better fixation by the deposition of new cartilage or bone at the points of friction and interaction between the fracture fragment, plate, and screw.

Treatment principles apply to individual cases but broad guidelines exist. The exact procedure followed may thus vary from patient to patient. Zone 2 injuries were traditionally explored via an open approach in the past, while injuries in zones 1 and 3 were subjected to conservative management with the help of imaging. This has now given way to a "no zone approach" where even zone 2 is treated with a conservative approach using CT angiography, Doppler, et cetera, thus reducing the morbidity and mortality associated with open approaches in neck trauma.

The paradigm of treating zone 2 injuries has thus shifted from the open approach to that adopted for zone 1 and 3 injuries, that is, monitoring with imaging and conservative management. This is only possible when soft signs are present as mentioned above. Apart from precipitating cardiogenic shock, the risk of septicemia and disseminated intravascular coagulation (DIC) is also increased manifold in the case of uncontrolled bleeding. Late complications such as neurological deficits and organ dysfunction are also common if bleeding is not managed in time. Surgical exploration must take into account the general condition of the patient and stabilization of vital parameters and blood volume.

The wound could then be explored immediately or an expectancy approach taken. Larger areas of laceration which are bleeding torrentially have to be managed with an emergency open exploration and repair of bleeding vessels. Other wounds might not be so obvious and deep injury has to be suspected. In these cases, the neck circumference should be monitored, and subcutaneous emphysema ruled out. Continued expansion in neck girth warrants a Doppler study and/or angiography to localize the bleed, and repair undertaken accordingly.

Furthermore, the larynx and trachea may be disrupted to various degrees and precipitate airway obstruction. Mucosal hematomas, vocal cord paralysis due to nerve damage or cricoarytenoid joint dislocation, impingement of fragments of cartilage from the larynx and trachea into the lumen, or complete separation of the larynx from the pharynx above or trachea below can all cause mechanical obstruction of the airway. Such injuries may preclude airway intubation and necessitate an open approach for wound exploration.

Open exploration of the neck and larynx, if and when necessary, is undertaken as soon as the patient is stabilized, preferably within 24–48 h. Delay beyond this interval makes surgical dissection challenging as tissue planes are distorted and the fracture fragments lose memory and elasticity.

6.2.3   A Tracheotomy

A tracheotomy must be done as low down in the neck as possible so that the stoma is well away from the site of potential repair. Injuries to the cervical spine are often an accompaniment of such trauma, and the neck cannot be extended as required for a tracheotomy. Thus it may have to be performed with the neck in flexion, which itself makes it a tedious and challenging procedure.

To minimize trauma due to instrumentation, a careful examination of the upper aerodigestive tract can be carried out with the help of a flexible bronchoscopy and esophagoscopy, as well as a direct laryngoscopy, either rigid or flexible.

The neck is then entered with a horizontal or collar incision, preferably over a natural skin crease, though neck outlines may be obliterated due to hematoma and subcutaneous emphysema. Bleeding may be negligible as early fibrosis sets into the muscle and tissue planes due to the soft tissue contusions in the neck.

6.2.4   The Laryngeal Skeleton Is Exposed

The laryngeal skeleton is exposed, and the injuries carefully assessed for displaced fragments, mucosal injuries, and cartilage loss or necrosis. Loose pieces of cartilage are best removed from the site as they serve no useful purpose and are potential sources of infection. Mucosal tears if large may be repaired with fine absorbable suture material and if small, may be left alone to get sealed on their own.

Fractures of the laryngeal skeleton must however be explored and repaired via an open approach. Fragments can be reduced and aligned with the main body of the larynx and secured with mini plates and screws. Wiring is another option but provides less stability and allows mobility of the fragments with swallowing movements. Open reduction and fixation of the laryngeal skeleton may also be achieved by suturing with 3.0 Vicryl, though plating has been reported to provide superior results. The latter may be an important constraint in resource poor regions that have to deal with laryngeal trauma.

6.2.5   Endolaryngeal Mucosal Trauma

Endolaryngeal mucosal trauma must be managed very delicately. Edges of viable mucosa must be approximated and sutured with fine, absorbable material without tension, and all areas of exposed cartilage covered properly. In the region of the anterior commissure, a keel may be kept temporarily to prevent the formation of adhesions and a consequent glottic stenosis. The subglottis and trachea should also be inspected for mucosal necrosis and cartilage exposure as this would predispose to tracheal stenosis. Stents may be used to prevent this but may not always be successful.

6.2.6   Local Repair

Local repair of a linear laryngeal fracture at the region of the vocal cords may be stabilized using a silicone sheet placed between the cords to prevent web formation. This may be kept in situ for about 6 weeks and removed through the neck incision without the need to open the larynx. In the case of a comminuted fracture, the laryngeal cartilage may be repaired, and a silicone stent or mold placed endolaryngeally for stabilization and removed after 8–12 weeks through an endoscopic approach after cutting the anchoring suture or wire. The duration of stenting depends on the gravity of the trauma and/or its reconstruction and also on individual preferences.

A *temporary stent* may be placed using a nasotracheal tube and kept in situ for 3–4 days to hold the reduction in place. Longer periods of stenting using such a method are not advised for fear of causing laryngomalacia. Devitalized segments of the trachea can be resected and end-to-end anastomosis carried out for lengths up to 6 cm.

6.2.7   Voice Rest

Voice rest is advised for up to a week, though cough, often violent, may potentially lead to disturbances in the reduction. Cough suppressants are not a good idea as they might cause secretions to stagnate and lead to surgical site infection. Instead pain, which is often the cause of cough in these cases, may be relieved with the help of adequate pain relief and sedation using agents such as fentanyl—an opioid analgesic.

6.2.8 Vigilance

Vigilance is maintained for signs of infection, which is always a looming threat in these injuries. Good antibiotic cover, adequate analgesia, anti-inflammatory medication, and anti-reflux agents must be included. Steroids should be avoided as far as possible in order to avoid superadded and opportunistic infection, though chondritis is best prevented with the help of steroids.

A good and almost invisible scar over the neck may be achieved by closing the surgical site in layers, with burying sutures in the subcutaneous plane using absorbable sutures and simple interrupted sutures on the skin using nonabsorbable suture material. The actual site of repair over the larynx is closed using overlapping layers of muscle and fascia.

In the absence of other injuries, early mobilization and decanulation may be carried out by downsizing and converting to a metal tracheotomy tube, which offers a chance for self-care and a quicker return to normalcy. The neck may be left open and covered with an antibiotic ointment, and the stay sutures can be removed by day 7 or so. A drain, if one has been used, is usually removed on the first postoperative day or as soon as the wound stops oozing.

6.2.9 Complications of Laryngotracheal Trauma

Complications of laryngotracheal trauma include granulations, granulomas, stenosis, and vocal cord immobility. The last one may be due to recurrent laryngeal nerve injury, subluxation or dislocation of the joint, hematoma in the joint space, or fibrosis of the joint. Direct laryngoscopy under general anesthesia helps to distinguish one from the other and also carry out a corrective procedure whenever possible. For example, a subluxation or dislocation may be rectified by anterior or posterior manipulation using a laryngeal retractor, flap elevator, or even the tip of the laryngoscope. Fibrosis of the joint is more difficult to treat, and in these cases an airway-widening procedure such as cordotomy or arytenoidectomy may be considered. Recurrent laryngeal nerve injury may be treated with a similar procedure if no spontaneous return of function occurs after a waiting period of 12 months. Stenosis at any level—supraglottic, glottic, subglottic, and tracheal—is a common and fearsome complication of laryngotracheal trauma, requiring complex surgery which may often produce unsatisfactory outcomes.

A popular method for treating tracheal stenosis is with the help of a balloon dilator, and this is known as endoscopic balloon dilatation (EBD). It may be done using a fiber optic endoscope with total intravenous anesthesia (TIVA) or a rigid direct laryngoscope as is the norm in suspension laryngoscopy with microsurgery. A tracheotomy may or may not be present. Many variations of this exist, such as simple balloon dilation with a Fogarty catheter, followed by steroid and/or mitomycin C injection, or using a "cutting" balloon dilator which has thin blades to make radial cuts through the scar tissue in addition to cutting, again followed by injection of either steroid or mitomycin C, and often both. It is generally considered safe and effective for early, soft or membranous stenosis though multiple sittings may be required. More than three attempts are considered an indication for open repair with resection—anastomosis or laryngotracheal reconstruction.

Complications, however, have been reported with EBD and include full thickness tears of the tracheal wall [6]. Underlying viscera may be exposed and may herniate into the tracheal lumen, or air may escape into the mediastinum and/or pleural space causing life-threatening problems on the operating table if not detected and treated promptly. Small tears may be sealed with fibrin glue, and slightly bigger ones which are only partial thickness could be sutured endoscopically. Positive airway pressure can be given to prevent viscera from prolapsing into the lumen. Silicone or metal stents may be placed through the endoscope to bridge the tear. Silicone stents are easier to remove at a later date when healing has taken place as they do not get incorporated into tissue, in contrast to a metallic stent. Thoracotomy and open repair of the tear may be required if contamination has occurred, for very large and complex tears and if the required expertise for endoscopic repair is not available.

6.2.10 Salivary Gland Trauma

In dealing with injuries to the salivary glands, primary repair is advocated but may not be feasible if more serious injuries demanding immediate attention are present. Utmost care must be taken to keep the area free from further contamination by administration of antibiotics and anti-inflammatory medications and drugs such as atropine or glycopyrrolate to reduce the production and flow of saliva. Steroids may be necessary when injury to nerves has occurred, especially to the facial or lingual nerves. Compression bandages and dressings and timely aspirations aided by postural drainage (if not contraindicated) help to "milk" the injured and "shocked" gland and avoid buildup of saliva in the vicinity of the wound. Salivary contamination may lead to problems with wound healing, for example, salivary fistula, and cause wound breakdown if primary surgical repair has been undertaken.

Salivary fistula is a dreaded sequel of trauma but may be a complication of other causes such as infection and neoplasia. The fistula may be external (glandular fistula) or open into the mouth (ductal fistula). The former is easier to manage with conservative measures such as antisialagogues, compression bandages, botulinum toxin, tympanic neurectomy, or the use of sclerosing agents such as sodium tetradecyl sulfate and hot water or hypertonic saline. Cyclandelate is also used by some practitioners. If unresponsive to medical measures, surgical removal of the entire gland and ductal structures may be required. This carries the risk of injury to major nerves such as the facial, lingual, and hypoglossal. If the gland is partially avulsed, it is better to remove it completely in order to avoid a salivary fistula. Duct repair can be done with monofilament fine absorbable sutures of 9.0 or 10.0 gauge using loupe magnification. Nerve repair is done with similar suture material of 6.0 or 7.0 size. A suction drain may be kept if necessary to minimize contamination with leaking saliva from gland remnants and removed once dry.

6.2.11 Vascular Trauma

If injury to the ICA in the neck is suspected, immediate exploration is warranted, and this may be facilitated by splitting the mandible (mandibulotomy) or swinging the temporomandibular joint laterally (mandibular subluxation). The ICA in the neck may be approached with a horizontal or collar incision to expose both sides or with a vertical incision along the sternocleidomastoid muscle if only unilateral exposure is required. Small tears in the ICA may be repaired primarily with fine monofilament sutures, taking care to coapt the edges of the vascular intima carefully in order to prevent the formation of microthrombi. Larger disruptions may require ligation, end-to-end anastomosis, and rerouting especially where part of the vessel needs to be resected. If a large segment of the vessel is missing, and rerouting so as to reduce the distance is also not possible, then grafting may have to be carried out. The graft material used may be taken from the patient's own body from another site using a vessel of similar caliber and other characteristics (autologous graft) or using cadaveric graft (homologous) or a synthetic material such as polytetrafluoroethylene (Gore-Tex alloplast graft). A bypass procedure may be performed if none of the above options are feasible, and a more proximal part of the vessel is connected to a terminal branch or a collateral vessel in the skull base or within the cranial cavity. This procedure may be performed only after confirming with a circle of Willis occlusion test which determines that the collateral vessels are functioning and robust.

6.2.12 Esophageal Trauma

Injury to the esophagus is a real but often underdiagnosed problem in neck trauma and is responsible for the majority of late morbidities such as tracheoesophageal fistula and mediastinitis. Contrast-enhanced esophagography poses radiation hazards and the risks of mediastinal spillage and contamination in the case of tears and perforations and is superseded by a direct visualization of the esophagus using rigid esophagoscopy under general anesthesia. This is conveniently undertaken at the time of the neck exploration and must be performed in order to avoid late surprises and a poor outcome. Plain X-rays of the neck are not beneficial in the diagnosis of esophageal injury as air leaks may be minuscule in the case of minor tears or in the presence of hematoma(s).

Tears of the esophagus in the cervical and thoracic segments may be easily missed on clinical examination. Even routine imaging with X-rays or CT scans may not reveal such injuries. Even if such an injury is suspected, the use of a contrast material to delineate the site is usually contraindicated for fear of causing mediastinitis and soft tissue cellulitis. A simple method to evaluate for tears of the esophagus is to fill the wound with warm sterile saline and inject air through the nasogastric tube, at the same time occluding the distal end of the esophagus by applying external pressure over the epigastrium at the level of the xiphisternum. This maneuver would cause air bubbles to appear in the wound, providing indirect evidence of a

Fig. 6.6 Esophageal stricture

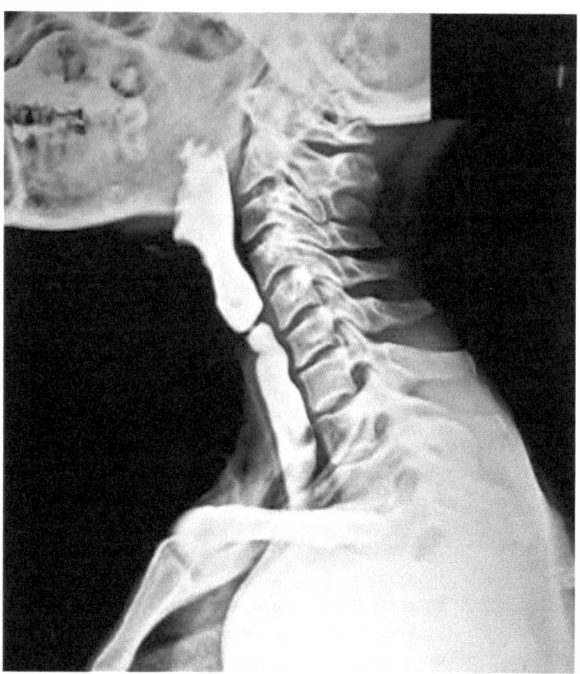

tear. Further investigation may then be done using a safe water-soluble contrast or directly with open surgical exploration. Esophageal tears may be repaired primarily in layers under direct vision using fine monofilament nonabsorbable sutures. The endotracheal tube cuff must be periodically deflated while repairing esophageal tears in order to minimize the risk of puncturing the ETT (endotracheal tube) cuff. Long-term complications of digestive tract injury include esophageal strictures, and these are more common in those who have suffered inhalation/ingestion trauma and/or airway instrumentation (Fig. 6.6).

6.2.13 Cervical Spine Trauma

Trauma to the neck involving the vertebral column or elements of the spinal cord and cervical cutaneous nerves may shear nerve fibers and lead to formation of a neuroma. This may present as a painful swelling in the neck and mimic other swellings such as a schwannoma or carotid body tumor. Thorough history taking should be able to pick out such a lesion and treat the same using medications given for neuralgic pain, such as methylcobalamin and carbamazepine or similar drugs. Control of the lancinating pain is more important than removal of such a swelling as communication with the spinal cord may cause minor or major disability ranging from paraparesis to quadriplegia.

6.2.14 Vocal Cord Lesions

Cricoarytenoid subluxation or dislocation causing vocal paralysis or asymmetry, if detected in time, may be treated primarily by closed reduction by gently manipulating with a laryngeal probe or the blade of a laryngoscope. Open reduction may be necessary in cases where fibrosis has occurred, but the results are poor. Usually by this time, adequate compensation has occurred, and further treatment is unnecessary. Intubation granulomas may be treated with a course of antibiotics, steroids, and anti-reflux medications. Botulinum toxin injection is an effective method of causing a temporary vocal cord paralysis and allowing the granuloma to resolve by minimizing or even eliminating vocal cord movement and friction.

A phonotraumatic lesion is first treated with speech therapy after a detailed speech assessment is made to identify faulty patterns of voice use. It is important to stress on vocal hygiene as a preventive measure to avoid a recurrence. Investigations include a videostroboscopy, perceptual voice analysis, and acoustic and aerodynamic measurements of voice by a trained speech and language therapist. Highly skilled professional voice users such as singers and actors require the services of a voice coach and counselor in addition to the above. A systematic regimen of voice hygiene and voice training is then instituted and must be strictly adhered to for best results. Psychological guidance or psychiatric consultation may be beneficial in highly stressed individuals. After a reasonable course of speech therapy, the vocal nodules are usually seen to disappear or shrink in size. Surgical excision is needed if problems continue or the nodules are long standing and large to begin with. Excision is carried out with microsurgical suspension laryngoscopy under general anesthesia using a medial microflap technique. A mucosal incision is taken at the medial edge of the vocal cord over the affected site, taking utmost care to avoid the most medial vibratory edge. A laryngeal elevator is used to dissect under the epithelial surface and enucleate the nodule with minimal effect upon the superficial lamina propria. Failure to do so or to simply "truncate" the nodule gives a suboptimal result as far as preservation of voice quality is concerned because this takes away a significant amount of normal superficial lamina propria as well.

Treatment of a vocal cyst is by surgical excision after a period of speech therapy has been tried. A vocal cyst is more deeply situated in the SLP (superficial lamina propria) and is therefore removed with the help of the lateral microflap trapdoor technique. A mucosal incision is made on the superior surface of the affected vocal cord toward the lateral border of the cyst and serves as the point of entry for submucosal dissection around the cyst, taking utmost care not to touch the unaffected SLP. After removal of the cyst, the mucosa snaps back into place due to elastic recoil, thus closing the incision. In this case also, "truncation" is avoided.

As far as the treatment of a vocal polyp is concerned, the protocol remains similar, that is, speech therapy followed by surgery in failed cases. As a vocal polyp has more or less left the boundaries of the SLP and is "dangling" over the mucosal epithelium, it may be gently delineated by medial traction and shaved off or "truncated" at its base, causing negligible effect upon the SLP. Restoration of voice quality is excellent in these cases provided voice therapy is instituted as part of the treatment process.

6.3   Best Practice Recommendations

- Digital tamponade, head elevation, stabilization of the cervical spine, oxygen by mask if available, and a penknife tracheotomy or cricothyrotomy in case of airway obstruction would be the minimum requirements for a safe transfer to hospital.
- The patient with a blunt or penetrating neck trauma must be managed expediently and methodically with open surgical exploration if necessary in the setting of the operating room. Selective exploration is however the current norm and is based on surveillance using imaging.
- Supraglottic, glottic, subglottic, or tracheal stenosis continues to be a dreaded complication of laryngotracheal trauma. Such an outcome is usually the result of suboptimal treatment of the primary trauma. Serial dilatations, resection and anastomosis, and laryngotracheal reconstruction are the methods of surgical treatment.
- The effect of iatrogenic airway trauma is ominous in more ways than one. The inflammation caused due to the intubation and the factors influencing it may continue unabated even when the need for intubation has ceased to exist and the patient has been extubated or decanulated.
- Gastroesophageal reflux disease (GERD) and laryngopharyngeal reflux (LPR), though not considered forms of trauma, are important predisposing and complicating factors. GERD often accompanies medical or systemic disease and is common in alcohol abusers, a risk group for suffering major trauma. LPR, on the other hand, may be a risk factor for laryngeal phonotrauma. Both may interfere with the administration of medical treatment, such as the use of antibiotics, analgesics and anti-inflammatory drugs, blood thinners, and so on. LPR in particular would need to be addressed prior to any kind of therapy given for laryngeal phonotrauma [7].

Conclusion

The neck is the abode of the life-sustaining organs of the body, the airway and food pipe. It also has the major blood vessels and nerves controlling the other organ systems and deserves special considerations in trauma, with ever increasing challenges and shifting paradigms of management.

References

1. Friedlander E, Pascual PM, Da Costa BJ, et al. Subluxation of the cricoarytenoid joint after external laryngeal trauma: a rare case and review of the literature. Indian J Otolaryngol Head Neck Surg. 2017;69:30.
2. Sachdeva K, Upadhyay A. Neck trauma: ENT prospects. Indian J Otolaryngol Head Neck Surg. 2017;69:52.
3. Chakraborty D, Das C, Verma AK, et al. Cut throat injury: our experience in rural set-up. Indian J Otolaryngol Head Neck Surg. 2017;69:35.
4. Poduval JD, Ali IE. Iatrogenic airway trauma: a systematic review. J Med Res. 2016;2(5):166–8.
5. Sanji RR, Channegowda C, Patil SB. Comparison of elective minimally invasive with conventional surgical tracheostomy in adults. Indian J Otolaryngol Head Neck Surg. 2017;69:11.
6. Heyes R, Cervantes SS, Matthaeus J, Jaroszewski D, Lott DG. Balloon dilation causing tracheal rupture: endoscopic management and literature review. Laryngoscope. 2016;126:2774–7.
7. Joshi AA, Chiplunkar BG, Bradoo RA. Assessment of treatment response in patients with laryngopharyngeal reflux. Indian J Otolaryngol Head Neck Surg. 2017;69:77.

Trauma to Eye and Orbit

7

Learning Objectives
- To learn the pathophysiology of trauma to the eye and orbit
- To understand the clinical implications of management of ocular and orbital trauma
- To remember the best practice recommendations in ocular trauma

7.1 Pathophysiology

7.1.1 The General Outline of Orbital Injury

The general outline of orbital injury is included in Chap. 5 along with injuries of the facial skeleton. This chapter is added to describe the finer points of injury to the orbit, globe, and eye in as much as a practicing otolaryngologist requires bearing in mind while treating facial trauma. Also, the relationship of the orbit to the paranasal sinuses makes many lesions including trauma in this region accessible to the endoscopic ENT surgeon.

The orbit is the bony enclosure in which the special sensory organ of vision is situated. The globe of the eye is made up of soft tissue with extremely intricate and sensitive neuroepithelium and the protective and conductive layers of the cornea, conjunctiva, lens, and aqueous humor. The extraocular muscles and ligaments, the nerves and blood vessels, and the lacrimal apparatus all surround the eye and help to serve its various functions. The average volume of the orbit in an adult is 30 ml, and nearly two thirds of this is composed of the muscles and nerves and soft tissues. An increase of just 4 ml in the volume of the globe is enough to cause proptosis of the eye.

The orbit is in the shape of a pyramid, with four sides, the base of which is in an anterior, lateral and inferior direction in the upper part of the facial skeleton, and the apex pointing toward and lying in the middle cranial fossa. It is thus related to the anterior cranial fossa superiorly, the maxillary antrum inferiorly, the infratemporal fossa infero-laterally, the middle cranial fossa supero-laterally, and the naso-ethmoid complex medially. As a result of this complex relationship, it is often involved in both head injuries and injuries of the temporal bone and facial skeleton.

The orbit has four walls—superior wall or roof, medial wall, inferior wall or floor, and lateral wall. Of these, the medial wall is the weakest as there is only a paper-thin bone, otherwise known as the lamina papyracea, separating the orbit from the ethmoid labyrinth. The floor is also relatively weak as the inferior orbital fissure and several foramina pass across it. The roof and lateral walls are comparatively thicker and stronger. The contents of the orbit are primarily soft tissue, namely, the globe and periorbita. These structures are also rich in vascular and nerve supply and house the special sensory organ of vision. In the event of trauma, tremendous pressure builds up inside the orbit within a short period of time due to the rupture of major vessels. This causes the contents of the globe to preferentially prolapse through the floor as a result of the dual effect of gravity and weakness, as compared to the medial wall. This is akin to the explosive rupture of a tennis ball in which the contents escape through the seams of the wall—in other words, a blowout. Thus fractures through the medial or inferior walls are known as orbital blowout fractures.

7.1.2 Blowout Fractures of the Orbit

Blowout fractures of the orbit, caused most frequently by direct frontal impact with an object about the size of a squash ball, such as a closed fist, lead to a sudden increase in the intraorbital pressure which in turn causes the relatively thinner and weaker orbital floor to give way and the intraorbital fat to prolapse into the maxillary antrum, producing the characteristic teardrop sign. The inferior rectus may also prolapse and be unable to retract back into the orbit as it gets entrapped by the bony fragments, leading to a trapdoor effect. The result is enophthalmos, facial asymmetry and external deformity, and diplopia due to restriction and imbalance of eye movements. A forced duction test would reveal entrapment of the muscle. If not treated in time, permanent enophthalmos may occur as the displaced fat undergoes necrosis and absorption.

Orbital fractures can permanently disrupt the shape of the orbit if not treated adequately and expediently, leading to expansion of the bony outline of the orbit. This, in association with mechanical disruption of the orbital soft tissue contents and their displacement, causes shrinkage of the constant volume in the orbit and results in enophthalmos [1]. The risk of enophthalmos is increased in the case of combined medial-inferior wall fractures of the orbit [2].

7.1.3 Injury to the Lacrimal Apparatus

Injury to the lacrimal apparatus is common in naso-orbito-ethmoid (NOE) fractures. If not detected promptly, permanent scarring of the canaliculi and/or nasolacrimal duct may occur, leading to complications such as epiphora and dacryocystitis.

Scarring in this region may cause the occurrence of an ectropion as well, making the epiphora worse. The type 3 NOE fracture, where the medial canthal ligament is completely avulsed from its attachment, is most likely to involve injury to the lacrimal apparatus as well.

Anatomically, injuries in this region can be assessed accurately by meticulous clinical examination including the patient's symptoms and signs, preferably with the help of an ophthalmologist. The following tests help to detect injury to the lacrimal drainage system:

1. *Primary Jones dye test*—A drop of fluorescein is instilled into the lower fornix of the conjunctiva and a cotton pledget moistened with topical anesthetic solution such as 4% lignocaine is placed just below the inferior turbinate of the ipsilateral nasal cavity. It is examined after 5 min for the presence of fluorescein, and the test is positive if it stains with fluorescein. This means that there is no injury to the lacrimal drainage pathway. If the test is negative, then the second step is done as follows.
2. *Secondary Jones dye test*—The fluorescein is flushed out from the conjunctival fornix by gentle irrigation, and the inferior canaliculus is cannulated and saline instilled through it. A new cotton pledget placed beneath the inferior turbinate is now examined for traces of fluorescein. The test is positive if fluorescein is found, signifying that the duct is patent but not functional due to reasons such as edema or neurological damage. If negative, then structural obstruction at the level of the punctum or canaliculus is suspected. Surgical repair may be needed to correct this.

7.1.4 The Second Cranial Nerve or Optic Nerve

The second cranial nerve or optic nerve emerges from the back of the globe, courses through the bony optic canal, and travels inward into the intracranial cavity. Shortly after coming out of the optic canals, the optic nerves of the two sides partially fuse to form the optic chiasma. The nerve fibers of the medial portions of either globe pass through the optic chiasma. Since the medial part of the retina of each eye is responsible for lateral vision, a lesion of the pre-chiasmatic portion of the optic nerve would impair vision in one eye alone, whereas a lesion in the post-chiasmatic portion of the nerve would cause a homonymous hemianopia, and a lesion of the chiasma, though rare, would cause a loss of both the lateral visual fields.

Injury to the orbit and optic canal can lead to the orbital apex syndrome, in which the 2nd, 3rd, 4th, 5th, and 6th cranial nerves are affected. These nerves except the 2nd (or optic nerve) may also be affected anywhere along their course as they pass through the superior orbital fissure.

A relative afferent pupillary defect (RAPD) or Marcus Gunn pupil is elicited using the "swinging flashlight test." When the light is shone on the unaffected eye, the pupil constricts, and when the light is moved to the opposite (affected) eye, the pupil of that eye also constricts but to a much lesser degree, thus appearing to dilate.

The reason for this is believed to be a lesion of the optic nerve on the affected side or retinal pathology in that eye or a lesion at the level of the optic chiasma. Thus, it is useful for the detection of optic nerve injury in case of trauma.

7.2   Clinical Implications

7.2.1   The Symptoms of Acute Trauma

The symptoms of acute trauma to the eye are pain and/or redness in the eye, blurring, diminution or loss of vision, double vision and facial disfiguration due to periorbital ecchymosis and edema, or swelling due to hematoma and prolapse of the globe. Subconjunctival hemorrhages, corneal abrasions or ulcerations, and hyphema may also be apparent. As time elapses and the hematoma is organized, the enophthalmos may become recognizable. Restriction of eye movement and disturbances of vision are the functional impairments caused by trauma.

Though ocular injury is commonly seen in the scenario of facial fractures, head injury and polytrauma, and may necessitate management by a specialist ophthalmologist, loss of function may rapidly ensue if appropriate and timely first aid is not administered by the primary trauma and emergency specialist. This includes a thorough history taking and examination, prompt management of corneal abrasions and/or hyphema, removal of conjuctival or corneal foreign bodies, and conjuctival/corneal burns.

7.2.2   The History

The history must include details about when and how the injury has occurred; what the possible injurious agent might have been; what the current symptoms of the patient are; whether any pre-existing eye disease, medical comorbidities, or allergies exist; if any medication has already been used; and when the patient last had anything to eat or drink, so as to determine whether general anesthesia can be administered in order to thoroughly explore the ocular injury and carry out appropriate management.

7.2.3   Physical Examination

Physical examination should consist of testing for reaction of the pupils to light, visual acuity by finger perception, finger counting and Snellen's chart, evaluation of eye movements, palpation for crepitus and exacerbation of symptoms which might suggest glaucoma, tonometry if possible, testing the fields of vision by perimetry, and fundoscopy to assess the status of the optic disc. A pale optic disc suggests optic nerve damage and must be dealt with expediently. A CT scan of the orbit and paranasal sinuses with coronal and axial cuts must be ordered at once, and impingement of the optic nerve by fragments of bone must be ruled out. All other cranial nerves must also be examined and neurological status determined.

7.2.4 Corneal Abrasions

Corneal abrasions may be examined by the instillation of a topical anesthetic, and any contaminating debris or foreign bodies must be removed gently. A cycloplegic agent such as homatropine 2% or cyclopentolate 1% can be used to relieve spasm of the ciliary muscle and allow the eye to rest. It may also prevent the onset of complications like iridocyclitis. Antibiotic in topical or oral form may be given according to the need of the patient. An eye patch with a gentle pressure bandage can be given for 24 h to provide tamponade and reduce edema. The treatment of hyphema may additionally require the administration of analgesics such as paracetamol and codeine, sedation, and head end elevation by 45° or so to reduce congestion in the eye.

7.2.5 Foreign Bodies

Foreign bodies may also be removed by initial application of a local anesthetic agent and systematic examination of the eye. Saline irrigation and using a soft cotton wipe or a 25 G needle to gently remove foreign bodies may also be tried. Corneal abrasions, if present, may be treated as described above. A protective eye patch to cover the cornea may be prescribed for up to a week in the acute phase of the injury. Chemical injuries may also be treated in a similar manner after copious irrigation with normal saline for at least an hour. The clinical examination and irrigation of the eye may be aided with the use of a conjunctival dilator if necessary.

7.2.6 The Initial Treatment of Orbital Blowout Fractures

The initial treatment of orbital blowout fractures is carried out by reduction of the fracture fragments. At the same time, any muscle that may be entrapped is released and returned to its normal position. The affected wall(s) of the orbit must be repaired by closed reduction if possible. This may be attempted for the medial wall by approaching through the nose with the help of an endoscope. For orbital floor fractures, open reduction is usually necessary, and the approach may be through a transconjunctival or subciliary incision to address the orbital floor directly or through the maxillary antrum using the Caldwell-Luc approach.

7.2.7 The Treatment of Established Enophthalmos

The treatment of established enophthalmos is carried out using an enophthalmic silicone wedge implant customized to fit the defect and restore lost volume to the globe and orbit. It should not be too large or too tight. The placement of an enophthalmic wedge implant is not without attendant risks, some of which are undue pressure on the optic nerve causing immediate loss of vision. Urgent re-exploration of the wound must be undertaken in such an event. There may also be increase in the intraorbital pressure due to the increase in volume of the orbital contents, leading to glaucoma. This may again cause blurring or loss of vision, and a lateral canthotomy must be done immediately to relieve the excessive pressure. If the implant is placed incorrectly, eye movements may be restricted, and too large an implant may result in persistent facial asymmetry and diplopia due to uncoordinated movements of the globes.

7.2.8   Optic Nerve Injury

Optic nerve injury may occur in the intraorbital, canalicular, or intracranial part. While the intraorbital part is approached via the sphenoid sinus and explored relatively more easily, the canalicular part may present challenges as it lies lateral to the sphenoid. Either the endoscopic or the open approach with the Lynch incision could be used. The bone over the canalicular portion must be inspected and fragments removed and the nerve fully decompressed by removing the overlying bone and slitting the nerve sheath, as trauma in this portion could cause obstruction of the communicating channels between the chiasmal cistern and the subarachnoid space, leading to edema over the nerve [3]. Where considerable edema of the nerve is evident, the sheath must be opened up to the tendinous ring of Zinn starting the incision of the orbital periosteum posteriorly and advancing anteriorly. This is believed to be particularly beneficial when there is no obvious fracture of this segment as evidenced by imaging, and the loss of vision is partial but is not justified when there is total loss of vision. The mechanism of action is by relief of pressure within the nerve sheath and reduction of edema and inflammation, and the results are promising even when a lot of time has elapsed between the trauma and its treatment.

For the otolaryngologist, all of the optic nerve is accessible with the rigid nasal endoscope, and this includes the apex of the orbit, the optico-carotid recess, the canalicular portion, and the optic nerve sheath, in that order. Optic nerve decompression for trauma should address a problem in any of these portions. To locate the orbital apex, a line parallel to the superior vertical ridge of the middle meatal antrostomy in the coronal plane should be followed till the meeting point of the posterior ethmoidal sinuses and the superior medial orbital wall. The optico-carotid recess may be identified at this junction, and the endoscope advanced medially towards the optic chiasma till the canalicular portion is reached. However, in order to do this, the bone over the optic nerve must be drilled away with the help of a diamond burr or removed carefully piecemeal using a periosteal elevator or bone curette. The presence of an Onodi cell, or posterior ethmoidal cell covering the orbital apex, causes the optic nerve to be exposed and dehiscent and may confuse the picture and make identification of the nerve at this point extremely difficult. The canalicular portion of the optic nerve is about a centimeter long, and the optic nerve sheath in this area merges with the dura mater of the brain. When this nerve sheath is incised, the optic nerve may be freed. At the same time, it is important to remember that in doing so the subdural space is also entered and is liable to result in a cerebrospinal fluid (CSF) leak, necessitating a CSF leak closure at the same time as the optic nerve decompression.

Optic nerve decompression is carried out with the help of general anesthesia. Local anesthesia to improve the surgical field may be provided with the use of Moffats's solution which is composed of 2 ml of 10% cocaine solution, 2 ml of 1:1000 adrenaline, and 1 ml of 2% sodium bicarbonate solution. Hypotensive anesthesia and a reverse Trendelenburg position can further make the surgery bloodless but are rarely necessary. Direct use of 1:1000 adrenaline on the nasal mucosa using neurosurgical patties, cotton pledgets, or ribbon gauze are other methods to enhance visibility during endoscopic surgical procedure. These must be used with caution and tight control by the anesthesia team to avoid myocardial ischemia and destabilization of the patient during surgery. Each and every infiltration and/or direct application of topical anesthetic or adrenaline must be done with the knowledge and approval of the anesthetist.

7.3   Best Practice Recommendations

- Blowout fractures of the orbit must be reduced and the globe realigned, but prior to this it is essential to make sure that no injuries to the lacrimal apparatus or retinal tears have occurred as these would necessitate attention first.
- If the extent of hypoglobus is less than 3 mm, it does not need any active surgical management. It may be left alone as the resulting deformity is not very obvious.
- In cases where the optic nerve sheath is compressed externally, the entire nerve sheath does not need to be opened along its length but only the cause addressed, such as a bone fragment or spicule or a hematoma on the nerve.

Conclusion
The eye and the orbit belong to the sister specialty of ophthalmology but hold an important territory for the otolaryngologist as well. Prompt treatment of injuries in this region is imperative in the event of facial trauma.

References

1. Clauser L, Galie M, Pagliaro F, Tieghi R. Posttraumatic enophthalmos: etiology, principles of reconstruction and correction. J Craniofac Surg. 2008;19:351–9.
2. He Y, Zhang Y, An JG. Correlation of types of orbital fracture and occurrence of enophthalmos. J Craniofac Surg. 2012;23:1050–3.
3. Sofferman RA. The recovery potential of the optic nerve. Laryngoscope. 1995;105(supplement 72):1–38.

Foreign Bodies in the Throat

8

Learning Objectives
- To learn the pathophysiology of foreign body ingestion and inhalation
- To understand the clinical implications of management of aerodigestive foreign bodies
- To remember the best practice recommendations in the treatment for foreign bodies

8.1 Pathophysiology

The larynx continues as the trachea at the level of the cervical vertebra C6, and the trachea divides into the right and left main bronchi at the level of the thoracic vertebra T4. The right main bronchus is shorter, wider, and more in line with the trachea and is therefore more likely to attract a foreign body. The cricopharyngeal sphincter at the level of C6—behind the cricoid ring of the larynx—is the narrowest portion of the digestive tract, and foreign bodies usually get impacted at this point. Once a foreign body has passed into the stomach, it generally passes into the lower gastrointestinal tract without the potential to cause further obstruction. The ileocecal junction is also a narrow portion of the digestive tract, and very rarely a foreign object may also get impacted here, especially if there is a diverticulum, stricture, or growth at this site.

8.1.1 Foreign Body (FB) Aspiration

Foreign body (FB) aspiration is seen more at the extremes of age due to a combination of poor reflexes and poor dentition. In children, two peaks are seen, one at 1–3 years and the second at 10–11 years due to the natural curiosity of exploring the

© Springer Nature Singapore Pte Ltd. 2018   153
J. Das, *Trauma in Otolaryngology*, https://doi.org/10.1007/978-981-10-6361-9_8

external environment, which is common to both these age groups. In the latter, play-fulness and the desire to show off are manifested in the tendency of older children to toss a coin or similar substance into the air and catch it in their mouth, with the accidental ingestion or inhalation of the article. Certain professions such as tailoring and dressmaking are also risk factors, and the risk is evident when workers hold a needle in their mouth from time to time while engaged in their task. Inebriated states and mental impairment are commonly associated with foreign body inhalation and impaction.

However, flipping a coin in the air and then trying to catch it in the mouth, habit-ually placing a needle between the teeth as certain persons in occupations such as dressmaking are wont to do, and even seemingly harmless habits such as nail biting are less common forms of foreign body entering the upper aerodigestive tract.

8.1.2   The Common Types of Foreign Body

The common types of foreign body are seeds, coins, and toy parts causing tracheo-bronchial and esophageal foreign bodies in children and dental plates, safety pins, bone, and food bolus in adults. An interesting and unfortunate instance of foreign body in the airway is a part of a tracheotomy tube especially that made of metal, which has broken off and slipped into the airway, sometimes with potential life-threatening implications [1].

The airway in small babies is especially prone to obstruction owing to the short and soft neck, a head size larger than the body size with the occipital area dispropor-tionately large, a soft and lax epiglottis, and a narrow subglottis with lax mucosa that is highly prone to edema. Respiratory distress in children is manifested by a rapid respiratory rate with or without fever, intercostal and subcostal retractions, alar flaring, and hypoxia as seen on pulse oximetry. Differential diagnoses include the common childhood diseases such as bronchiolitis, croup, pneumonia, and asthma. But no time must be lost in trying to reach a diagnosis, and the airway must be secured right away.

8.1.3   The Clinical Features

The clinical features are most importantly a positive history of foreign body visual-ized entering or being inserted into the body, which may be available in roughly 80% of cases, with or without choking followed by paroxysmal coughing, a hoarse cry, restlessness, dyspnea, stridor, and exhaustion from breathing against resistance as the child settles down due to fatigue and adaptation. Tachypnea, tachycardia, and cyanosis may be present in advanced cases where the foreign body has caused sig-nificant obstruction and hypoxia.

Foreign bodies in the aerodigestive tract in children and babies may not be accompanied by a positive history or evident on examination. Children decompensate very rapidly and may even collapse as a result of respiratory compromise due to airway obstruction. While an airway foreign body is the obvious culprit, respiratory obstruction could also result from a large foreign body in the food passage as well. Many a time, the child is in a very critical condition, and intervention has to be immediate and based on the physical condition of the patient and not necessarily on the diagnosis, which might be done after stabilization of the airway crisis.

8.1.4 Diagnostic Dilemmas

Diagnostic dilemmas may occur due to the absence of a positive history and the presence of coughing, choking, or wheezing, in which case the differential diagnoses would include croup (laryngotracheobronchitis) or bronchial asthma. A sudden onset of wheezing, especially unilateral, should settle the clinical suspicion. Unexplained fever may be due to persistent or recurrent pneumonitis due to lobar pneumonia caused by a retained foreign body. In the presence of an upper respiratory tract infection (URTI) inhalation is more common due to mouth breathing and coughing. A change in the cry to hoarse or stridulous, excessive salivation, gurgling sounds, and refusal to eat should immediately arouse suspicion of a foreign body. The risk of respiratory failure is high in infants as they have a very low respiratory reserve, narrow airway, high peripheral airway resistance, and a higher basal metabolic rate (BMR) and oxygen consumption per minute. There is also more loss of heat with a rapid respiratory rate, which leads to dehydration, and the functional residual capacity (FRC) of the lungs is reduced.

The clinical signs may evolve with the first signs which are caused due to change in the air flow in the lungs. An audible click or fluttering noise may be heard due to the movement of the foreign body in the tracheal air stream. The chest movements may be pronounced. The site of impaction may be clinically estimated by the occurrence of severe or total respiratory obstruction, in which case the foreign body is more likely to be in the larynx. A clicking or fluttering sound may be heard even in cases of near obstruction. If the foreign body is in the carina, there may be shifting signs. A unilateral expiratory wheeze may be heard when the foreign body is in the bronchus, and when it is in a lung lobe, there is reduced air entry and conducted breath sounds.

8.1.5 The Reaction of the Bronchial Mucosa

The reaction of the bronchial mucosa is an intense inflammation if the foreign body is organic or vegetable matter. This is due to the presence of lipoid. It leads to mucosal swelling, inflammatory exudates, and the production of granulation tissue. The risk of impaction is increased and bronchial obstruction may occur, resulting in atelectasis and lung abscess. The risk of thromboembolism is also increased. In the case of a dry vegetable foreign body, very rapid obstructive changes may occur due to mucosal irritation and hygroscopic swelling of the material causing a rapid onset of collapse or atelectasis of the distal lung. The presence of florid granulation tissue causes hemoptysis. Metal foreign bodies cause less irritation and a slower progression to complete obstruction. Inert or smooth foreign bodies cause minimal or no reaction and no risk of pneumonia unless the size is large. Large esophageal foreign bodies can compress the trachea and cause respiratory obstruction, whereas sharp esophageal foreign bodies may result in a tracheoesophageal fistula which may also cause respiratory symptoms. Pain at the root of neck and larynx may be present in some cases.

Important prognostic indicators are the age of the patient, type of foreign body—whether vegetable or inorganic, sharp, or rounded—the site of impaction (in glottis or subglottis), the interval between entry and removal, the skill of the anesthetist, and the availability of proper equipment and instrumentation.

8.1.6   Foreign Bodies in the Esophagus

Foreign bodies in the esophagus may cause various degrees of injury as follows:

1. *First degree*—mucosal abrasions, edema, or superficial tears
2. *Second degree*—partial thickness tears with bleeding and thinning of the muscular wall and small, complete tears without contamination of the surrounding areas
3. *Third degree*—full thickness tears of the wall with mediastinitis, pneumothorax, air embolism, or abscess formation

Symptoms of esophageal perforation are pain at the root of the neck (cervical esophagus) or between the shoulder blades (thoracic esophagus). Sometimes the pain may be in the epigastrium (mimicking gastritis) or even referred to the left upper limb (mimicking angina pectoris). Surgical emphysema over the neck or upper chest wall may be evident from progressive swelling and crepitations in these regions.

Foreign bodies in the aerodigestive tract are potentially life-threatening and are responsible for approximately 3000 deaths per year in acute cases due to respiratory obstruction. In chronic cases complications of retained FB include chronic lung disease and hypoxic brain damage due to delayed removal of the FB to relieve respiratory obstruction.

The mnemonic "LEMON"—look out, evaluate (the situation swiftly), (determining the) Mallampati score, (ruling out and relieving) obstruction, and (assessment of the) neck—is a useful guide to the management of acute airway obstruction in children, including that caused by a foreign body.

8.1.7 Radiological Features

Radiological features are very useful in the detection of foreign bodies but may also be misleading. Correct X-rays must be ordered, for example, spanning the nasopharynx and pelvis in indicated cases. The neck must be extended and anteroposterior (AP) and lateral views must be taken. The AP views must be in both inspiration and expiration. A chest X-ray in the lateral decubitus position or a chest X-ray posteroanterior (PA) view may be required in the case of inhaled foreign bodies to assess the lung fields and pulmonary status. An air bronchogram may be seen in cases where bronchial impaction has occurred. A CT scan may be required in rare cases, as well as isotope scans to look for changes in the ventilation/perfusion ratio. A diagnostic endoscopy is considered the gold standard.

Changes seen on X-ray are air trapping and mediastinal shift. In obstructive emphysema the mediastinum is seen to shift to the normal side and in atelectasis to the obstructed side. In lobar pneumonia consolidation without mediastinal deviation is seen. Arachidic bronchitis refers to the peculiar pattern seen on a chest X-ray due to bronchial irritation caused by a vegetable foreign body. The inflammatory reaction is so intense and widespread that it looks like the web of a spider, hence the name "arachidic," derived from "arachnid." Plain X-rays may be positive in 90% of cases but normal in about 10%. X-ray manifestations increase after 24 h, and therefore imaging may have to be repeated if required. In about 20% of cases, there is no positive history and no radiological signs. The right bronchus is more susceptible to impaction compared to the left bronchus as it is shorter, wider, and straighter.

Esophageal foreign bodies are easily detected if they are radiopaque. Contrast studies may show a filling defect in the case of a radiolucent foreign body. There is also widening of the prevertebral soft tissue shadow on lateral X-ray of the neck. Air may be seen in the soft tissues of the neck, as also an air pocket in upper esophagus in case of bolus obstruction.

The prevertebral soft tissue widening is considered significant if it exceeds two thirds of the body of the vertebra at that level or an absolute dimension of 7 mm at the level of the C1–C2 vertebra, 14 mm at the level of the C3–C4 vertebra, and 21 mm at the level of the C5–C6 vertebra (Fig.8.1).

The sites of impaction are usually the natural points of narrowing of the esophagus at 15 cm (cricopharyngeal sphincter), 25 cm (crossing of the arch of aorta), 27 cm (crossing of the left main bronchus), and 40 cm (entry of esophagus into the stomach at the level of the diaphragm) from the incisor teeth. The narrowing is increased due to mass lesions, either benign or malignant. Also, peristalsis weakens with age and sensations are decreased. Thus, the risk of impaction is greater in the elderly, and they are vulnerable to recurrent foreign body impaction due to the above reasons. In recurrent bolus obstruction, motility disorders must be ruled out by videofluoroscopy.

Imaging for foreign bodies in the oral cavity or oropharynx is not indicated and is therefore not very popular, as the bony shadow of the mandible tends to obscure any foreign body that might be present in this region.

Fig. 8.1 Prevertebral
widening with linear
radiopacity

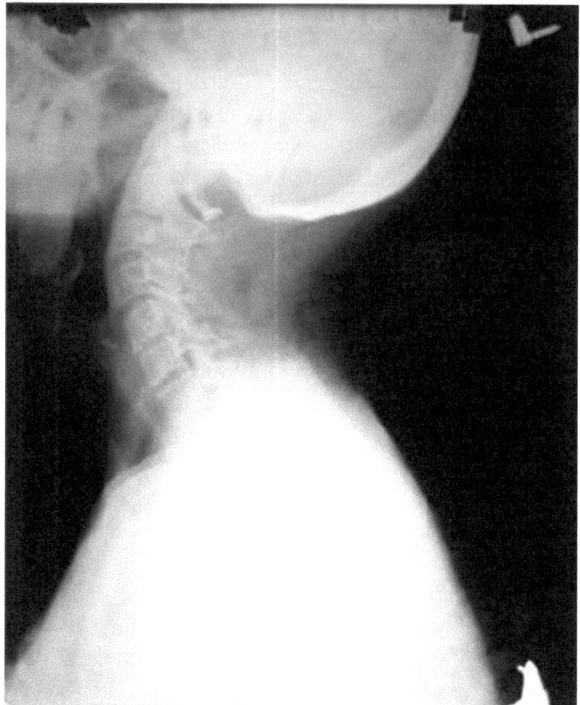

Sometimes it may be extremely challenging to determine the location of the foreign body, especially if it is small and radiolucent, and presents with symptoms common to both the airway and the food pipe. For example, if a small cartilaginous fish bone has been ingested, it could cause mucosal tears in the gastrointestinal tract and result in vomiting of blood-stained secretions. These refluxed and regurgitated contents may be aspirated and cause coughing, choking, or frank respiratory distress. Alternatively, such a foreign body could be aspirated into the airway and cause choking and coughing, which when occurring after a meal could provoke irritation in the digestive tract and lead to vomiting. Such confusion arises more commonly in the case of babies and young children. The only way to proceed would be to do a diagnostic endoscopy—a rigid bronchoscopy preferably using a ventilating bronchoscope, followed by a rigid esophagoscopy after securing the airway with an endotracheal tube.

8.2   Clinical Implications

8.2.1   The Simplest Procedure

The simplest procedure to relieve airway obstruction is the "head tilt and chin lift," which helps to align the oropharyngeal and laryngeal airways and relieve the upper airway obstruction to some extent. In suspected foreign body aspiration, a "jaw thrust" is useful. Chest or back thumps are also useful in expelling foreign bodies from the airway of small children whereas the standard Heimlich maneuver can be tried in older children and adults. The Heimlich maneuver and back thumps may be successful, but the risk of impaction is also increased. Procedures such as postural drainage and digital manipulation of FB may dislodge the FB and cause total respiratory obstruction.

Failure with any of the above methods calls for more definitive measures such as the introduction of a supraglottic device in the form of a laryngeal mask airway or endotracheal intubation if possible. In foreign body aspiration, this is often difficult or even impossible to perform, and recourse must be made toward direct visualization of the airway with a fiber optic bronchoscope or making a surgical airway in the form of a cricothyrotomy or tracheotomy.

8.2.2 Advances in Anesthesia

Advances in anesthesia have made spontaneous breathing possible with inhalation anesthesia using a ventilating bronchoscope. Alternatively, induction may be done with sodium pentothal, muscle relaxation with succinylcholine, and oxygenation with face mask.

The larynx may be sprayed with 4% Xylocaine, oxygenation with face mask repeated, the bronchoscope introduced, and jet ventilation administered. The apnea technique, popular in the earlier era, is now outdated and considered extremely risky. It involves performing the procedure rapidly within a span of 4 min, which is the upper limit for brain hypoxia to occur. Even in expert hands, mortality with this procedure is very high, almost close to 100 percent, and understandably so, very few surgeons now perform this hazardous procedure except in poorly equipped settings. Total intravenous anesthesia (TIVA) and a laryngeal mask airway (LMA) are other options for foreign body removal.

8.2.3 The Prerequisites of a Safe Procedure

The prerequisites of a safe procedure would be to:

1. Check all instrumentation thoroughly.
2. Preferably do practice passes through a mannequin or dummy (simulation).
3. Introduce the endoscope with the right hand.
4. Stabilize the upper teeth with the left hand.
5. Use the suction and forceps with the right hand while the endoscope is transferred to the left hand.

In esophagoscopy, endotracheal intubation may be undertaken, but an emergency tracheotomy may sometimes be required. In long-standing cases, preoperative antibiotics and chest physiotherapy may be required in addition. If respiratory distress is absent, an elective procedure may be done after relevant investigations. Contrast studies with a water-soluble dye such as Gastrografin may be done safely in the case of a suspected esophageal injury.

8.2.4   Visualization

Visualization may be difficult during bronchoscopy. Rigid endoscopy is always preferable to flexible endoscopy in the removal of a foreign body because of better control of the airway. A foreign body of any size or shape can be managed efficiently. There is better illumination, natural color, and wide-angle viewing, and instrumentation is possible for suction and biopsies of suspicious lesions if any, along with the removal of the foreign body.

The lobar bronchi on the right side must be examined first. The holes of the bronchoscope must be kept unobstructed at all times. In esophagoscopy, the cricopharynx, mid-esophagus, and lower esophagus must be thoroughly examined. The region of the hypopharynx may be especially tricky to visualize and requires specific procedures to avoid missing a foreign body [2]. Though these have been described for the detection of hidden malignancies, a knowledge of the same would help in the detection of small foreign bodies or those with almost the same color as the mucosa, for example, dentures. A CT scan may sometimes be necessary and specific regions of the hypopharynx meticulously searched (Figs. 8.2, 8.3, 8.4, 8.5, 8.6, 8.7).

Fig. 8.2 CT hypopharynx—axial view; valleculae

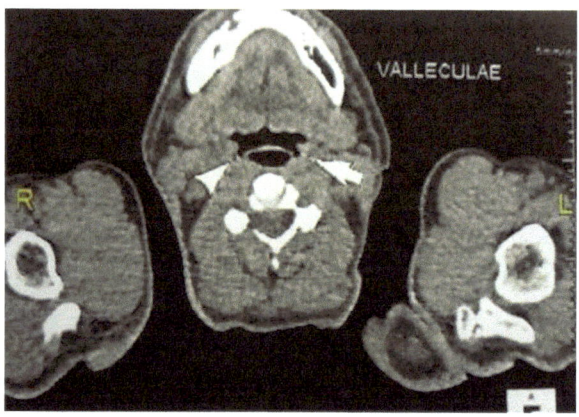

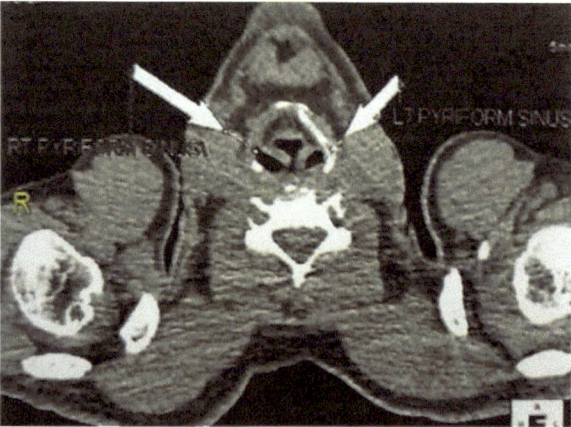

Fig. 8.3 CT hypopharynx—axial view; pyriform sinuses

Fig. 8.4 CT hypopharynx—
coronal view; valleculae

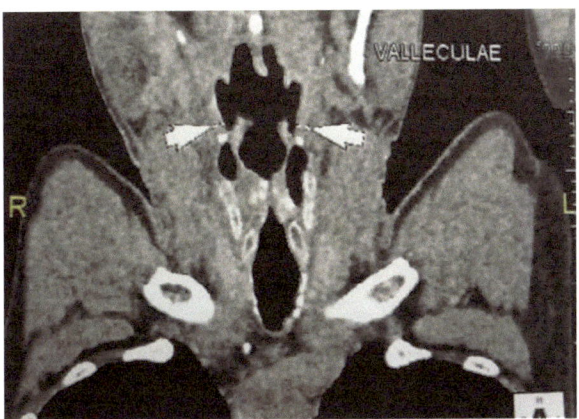

Fig. 8.5 CT hypopharynx—
coronal view; pyriform
sinuses

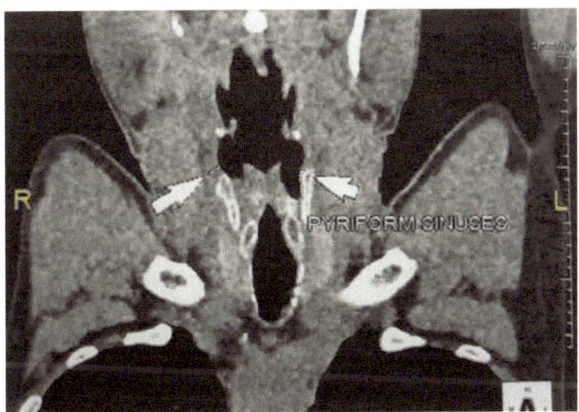

Fig. 8.6 CT hypopharynx—
sagittal view; epiglottis and
vallecula

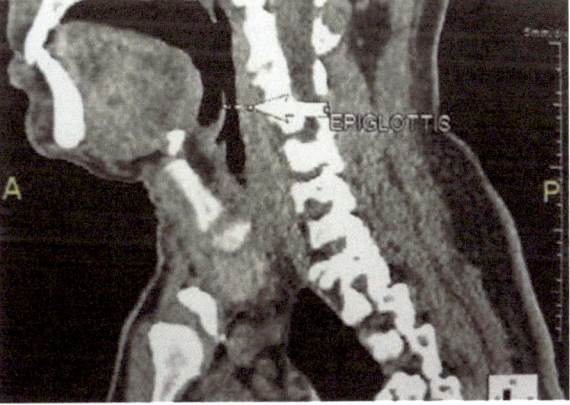

A rigid hypopharyngoscopy and esophagoscopy followed by nasopharyngoscopy, laryngoscopy, and bronchoscopy would help to confirm the presence or absence of foreign bodies. A second look must be taken to ensure completeness of removal and to rule out aspiration of pus or mucus. If the procedure is

Fig. 8.7 CT
hypopharynx—sagittal
view; pyriform sinus

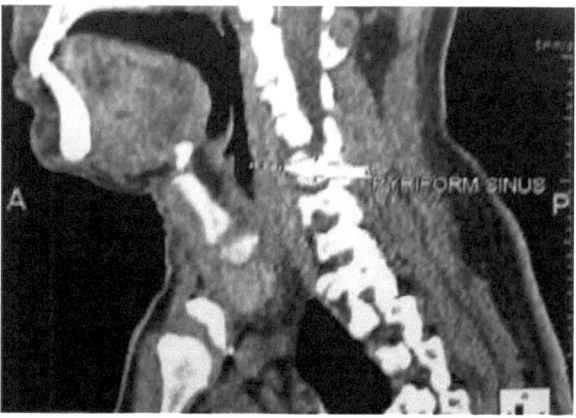

prolonged, intravenous (IV) corticosteroids must be administered in addition to antibiotics, and a nasogastric tube is also inserted and the patient kept nil per oral for 24–72 h.

8.2.5 Points to be Noted During the Endoscopy

Points to be noted during the endoscopy are the characteristics of the foreign body, the appearance of the mucosa, the nature of secretions, mass lesions if any, compression or collapse of the lung, mobility or blunting of the carina, and the appearance of washings, suction, and any biopsies that are taken.

8.2.6 Complications of Endoscopy

Complications of endoscopy include laryngeal spasm; mucosal edema; hemorrhage; damage to teeth, lips, and cervical spine; bronchial rupture or pneumothorax; cardiac arrhythmias; and esophageal perforation.

8.2.7 Complications of Esophageal FBs

Complications of esophageal FBs are respiratory obstruction if the retained foreign body is large, and perforation in the case of sharp foreign bodies, with or without formation of an abscess in the neck. Cases of severe impaction may require thoracotomy or even gastrotomy, after pushing the foreign body into the stomach.

Small or partial thickness tears may be managed conservatively, but a nasogastric tube must be inserted for 7–10 days to maintain nutrition and prevent mediastinal complications. Larger tears must be explored by an open approach such as neck exploration or thoracotomy.

Foreign bodies may get impacted in the soft tissues of the head and neck or inside the spaces and crevices of the upper aerodigestive tract in cases of facial injuries. A preliminary clinical examination must rule out this possibility prior to fixation of facial fractures with wiring or plating, especially if the patient is not in a position to provide historical details. Vomiting, bleeding, cough, hemoptysis, and respiratory distress are common complications of foreign bodies thus missed. Removal of the fixation by cutting the wires, and an elective tracheotomy to safeguard the airway, must be undertaken in order to search for such foreign bodies.

8.3   Best Practice Recommendations

- Calcification of the thyroid cartilage may start as early as the second decade of life and is seen first in the posterior aspect (border) of the thyroid cartilage. Such areas of calcification can be mistaken for a foreign body when a suggestive history is present. A diagnostic esophagoscopy is advised in symptomatic cases.
- Sometimes a panendoscopy (this includes a bronchoscopy, laryngoscopy, nasopharyngolaryngoscopy, and esophagoscopy—preferably in this order in view of the likelihood of migration of the foreign body) is necessary in order to localize and remove the missing object.
- Prevention of foreign body aspiration may be done by increasing awareness and education, preventing access, setting a good example, maintaining a high index of suspicion for prompt treatment, and prevention of complications due to retained foreign bodies. Simple passage of balloon catheters, enzymatic dissolution, and unscientific procedures should be strictly avoided.

Conclusion
Foreign body impaction, both by ingestion and inhalation, is a common occurrence for the otolaryngologist and can pose life-threatening injuries. It may be considered a form of internal injury which is invisible and presents in an indirect manner but must be expediently managed.

References

1. Poduval J, Benazir F, Ninan P. Pneumopericardium – an unusual complication of broken tracheostomy tube presenting as foreign body trachea. J Laryngol Voice. 2014;4:32–5.
2. Thakur P, Poorey VK. Manoeuvres to improve endoscopic visualization of hypopharynx. Indian J Otolaryngol Head Neck Surg. 2017;69:93–6.

Case Scenarios

9

Learning Objectives
- To present real-life situations in trauma for different levels of practitioners as a form of problem solving exercises
- To present a quick recap and assess the general knowledge of important facts pertaining to trauma in the head, face, and neck.

9.1   Case Scenarios by Region

9.1.1   Ear

1. A 10-year-old child complains of ear pain and impaired hearing after being involved in a fist fight 2 days earlier. He is a known case of allergic rhinitis. Examination reveals a soft fluctuant swelling over the right pinna, and the eardrum has a dark discoloration. Tuning fork tests show conductive hearing loss on both sides. Discuss the further management of this patient.
   (a) Diagnosis
       Trauma to external and middle ear with allergic rhinitis and bilateral conductive hearing loss.
       A fist fight suggests a blunt trauma to the head and face from the frontal or, in this case, lateral aspect. The pain and hearing impairment are due to this impact. The soft swelling over the pinna is probably an auricular hematoma. The discoloration of the drum is due to a hemotympanum, but the opposite ear needs to be examined carefully to rule out otitis media with effusion, which is common in allergic rhinitis. This explains the bilateral conductive loss.
   (b) Investigations

DNE—diagnostic nasal endoscopy must be done to determine the status of the allergic rhinitis, the presence of hypertrophied adenoids, polyps, or structural anomalies.

PTA—pure tone audiometry must be carried out to determine the quality, extent, and symmetry of the hearing impairment, coupled with an impedance audiometry.

CT temporal bone—this would establish beyond doubt the possibility of a longitudinal or otic-capsule-sparing type of temporal bone trauma but is not mandatory.

The status of the facial nerve must be determined and documented at every review.

Lab tests must exclude common conditions such as anemia, diabetes, and bleeding disorders from the point of view of incipient surgical intervention and overall prognosis.

(c) Treatment

Evacuation of the hematoma by deroofing/window operation.

Control of allergic rhinitis.

Close follow-up until hemotympanum subsides. Serial audiograms should exclude an ossicular discontinuity or fixation due to fibrosis and ankylosis.

2. A 35-year-old housewife presents with acute-onset earache and difficulty in hearing after a domestic quarrel in which her husband slapped her. Examination of the ear reveals a few blood clots deep in the ear canal. Tuning fork tests suggest a mild conductive loss on the same side. How would you manage this patient?

(a) Diagnosis

Traumatic perforation of tympanic membrane with conductive hearing loss.

This is a case of blast trauma with transmission of a pressure wave from the environment into the vibrating apparatus of the ear. It causes a shearing force across the surface of the tympanic membrane with rupture of its vessels and minor bleeding which stops spontaneously. Sometimes ossicular discontinuity may occur due to dislocation or subluxation of the ear ossicles. Very rarely such an impact might even cause sensorineural damage and irreversible hearing loss. Tinnitus may be a significant accompanying symptom and could be temporary or permanent.

(b) Investigations

EUM—an examination under the microscope would help to remove the blood clots and determine the size and shape of the perforation. Such a perforation is usually moderate in size and elliptical in shape, with irregular or jagged edges.

PTA—a pure tone audiometry must be done to confirm the nature and severity of the hearing loss. A patch test would help to further confirm this. For this, a baseline audiometry is first performed, followed by the placement of a small piece of moistened sterile cigarette paper to seal the perforation and repeating the audiogram. Correction of the hearing and abolition of tinnitus, if any, would prove the diagnosis of traumatic perforation.

A psychiatry consultation is advisable in order to deal with the issue of marital stress and spousal abuse.

(c) Treatment

In most cases, the patch test is not only confirmatory but also therapeutic and would help to seal the perforation. Because this is a fresh injury, fibroblasts grow from the edges of the perforation and facilitate healing. This normally takes up to 3–4 weeks but is hastened by the patch which acts as a scaffold.

Even if a patch test is not done, the edges of the perforation should be examined carefully under the microscope and may be found to be curled inward. These are then everted under vision so that regeneration of epithelium can take place in an outward direction. Otherwise, squamous epithelium from the ear canal may grow into the middle ear cavity. Healing then occurs naturally over the next 3–4 weeks. Antibiotics are usually not necessary. The ear must be kept dry and entry of water should be avoided. Topical eardrops are optional and not usually required or even recommended.

3. A 50-year-old man is brought to A&E in an unconscious state and bleeding from the left ear as result of a motor vehicle accident. The GCS is 3/15, and on local examination the auricle is found to be almost completely severed from the skull. The edges are now oozing and the wound is covered with dirt and grime. Battle's sign is absent. What would be the line of management for this patient?

(a) Diagnosis

Head injury [with or without polytrauma] with avulsion of auricle.

This patient has suffered a head injury, and therefore attention must be drawn to this first before anything else. It is imperative to ensure that the ABCs of acute trauma are in place, that is, the patient has a patent airway, is breathing spontaneously, and is not actively bleeding either externally or internally—in that order.

The head injury in this case is likely to be severe, and airway compromise would be imminent. This, and the fact that the GCS is below 8/15, necessitates immediate endotracheal intubation. Furthermore, if the patient is not breathing spontaneously, he must be connected to a ventilator as soon as possible. The vital parameters must be optimized by the insertion of an intravenous line, urinary catheter and nasogastric tube, and any other means for artificial life support if required. The primary and secondary survey must exclude injury to other systems such as the thorax, abdomen, pelvis, and lower limbs. Only after this is the ear wound assessed. The ear injury in this case is an avulsion of the auricle. The middle and inner ear, as well as the facial nerve, are difficult to assess at this juncture.

(b) Investigations

A plain CT scan of the brain must be arranged expediently and the extent of intracranial injury assessed so that evacuation of a hematoma, if any, may be undertaken as soon as the patient is stabilized. Lab investigations must be sent accordingly and would at the minimum include a complete hemogram with coagulation profile, blood gases, serum electrolytes, and renal function tests. Injuries to other systems would require appropriate imaging such as X-rays, ultrasound, and Doppler studies.

(c) Treatment

Local treatment for the auricle avulsion is carried out only after the patient is stabilized. Such an extensive avulsion is rarely viable if sutured back in place, but primary repair may be carried out in the absence of facilities for a microvascular flap repair. The wound is copiously irrigated with saline and dilute hydrogen peroxide to get rid of blood clots, dried crusts, dirt, and other contaminants and the wound carefully examined to rule out traces of embedded materials like glass, metal, or wood. Burns, if any, should be carefully handled and the edges of the wound freshened or resurfaced. Exposed cartilage or loss of tissue should be documented. Primary suturing of the wound edges is then performed with fine nonabsorbable monofilament or polyfilament material. Daily dressings and reviewing the progress of the wound are essential, as are antibiotics and other appropriate medications. Tetanus toxoid prophylaxis is advised.

4. A 40-year-old female executive presents with severe ear pain and fullness in the right ear after returning from an overseas trip. She also has a cold and some difficulty in following conversations. Examination shows an intact eardrum with bubbles and a mild conductive deafness on the affected side. The nasal septum is deviated to the same side and the mucosa is congested. Discuss the management of this patient.

(a) Diagnosis

Ear barotrauma with acute middle ear effusion.

This is a case of barotrauma following descent during a flight. Normally, the Eustachian tube equalizes the air pressure in the middle ear cavity with the atmospheric pressure by opening and allowing air escape from the middle ear as the external pressure rises. During a cold or due to mechanical obstruction such as a deviated nasal septum, the Eustachian tube becomes dysfunctional and fails to open. This leads to buildup of air in the external ear and nasopharynx and pain due to this increased air pressure. There may also be minor hemorrhages over the tympanic membrane leading to persistence of the pain even up to a few hours or days after the flight. The air in the middle ear cavity is absorbed, creating a vacuum and drawing intracellular fluid into the extracellular compartment, that is, the middle ear cavity. This is the reason for the appearance of bubbles behind an intact drum and the feeling of fullness in the ear. The presence of fluid also causes a mild hearing loss of conductive type.

(b) Investigations

This is a clinical diagnosis based on history and examination and generally does not require extensive investigations. An impedance audiometry may be done to confirm the presence of fluid and a pure tone audiometry to confirm conductive hearing loss, but both are unnecessary and uncomfortable for the patient in the presence of pain and fullness. These, and appropriate lab tests, would only be required if the patient does not respond to the initial treatment, in which case the diagnosis could be reexamined.

(c) Treatment

Immediate symptomatic relief must be given to the patient in the form of decongestant nose drops and avoidance of nose blowing. Painkillers may be prescribed if necessary. Antibiotics are usually not required, either systemically or topically. The ear must be kept dry to prevent infection from the ear canal. The patient must be counseled about the gradual resolution of the problem over the next few days and for the fullness to subside completely along with the restoration of normal hearing. Steroids may be given if absolutely required and if the patient expects or demands a rapid recovery in order to cope with the nature of her work. The side effects of such therapy must be explained to the patient. The nose must be examined carefully after a few days to exclude local pathology. Assessment of the nasal septal deviation may necessitate septal surgery at a later date. The patient must be warned about similar occurrences during future flights and asked to use nasal decongestant drops a few days before such trips. Active swallowing and sucking on lozenges during descent are also advised.

5. A 60-year-old schoolteacher suffers a mugging attack and falls unconscious. He is brought to the hospital by passersby and is found to have a GCS of 12/15, with bleeding from the left ear and a facial paralysis on the same side. There are no other injuries anywhere on the body. What would be the line of management of this patient?

(a) Diagnosis

Head injury with temporal bone fracture with lower motor neurone facial paralysis.

This is most likely a concussion injury due to a blow to the back of the head. The increased age and a probable lateral impact have caused the predominantly ear trauma. There is probably a temporal bone fracture of the otic-capsule-violating type, with laceration of the external auditory canal skin as well. The facial nerve palsy is immediate and complete.

(b) Investigations

A plain CT scan of the brain with temporal cuts would help confirm both the absence of an intracranial bleed and the presence of the temporal bone fracture. Otoscopy would confirm the loss of continuity of the external canal wall skin, with or without injury to the tympanic membrane and/or a CSF (cerebrospinal fluid) leak. Lab tests must be done to exclude anemia, diabetes, and other common systemic illnesses.

(c) Treatment

Antibiotics and steroids by the parenteral route must be started at once, along with adjuvant therapy such as antacids and anti-inflammatory agents. Once the absence of a CSF leak has been confirmed, the ear canal must be gently but snugly packed with an antibiotic-steroid ointment to prevent the development of canal stenosis. Alternatively, a stent coated with antibiotic and steroid may also be inserted. However, an overt CSF leak or a suspicion about the same would warrant the addition of Diamox (acetazolamide) by nasogastric tube as long as the patient remains unconscious. In such a case, packing of the ear canal should be avoided and the patient given a slight head elevation with the affected ear (side of head) turned upward (toward the opposite side). The leak should gradually subside with this approach. Straining and nose blowing must be avoided and stool softeners added as the patient is likely to develop constipation. The facial nerve must be monitored and eye care and facial physiotherapy started immediately. Return of function suggests a neurotmesis or axonotmesis, but its absence even after 3 weeks suggests a complete or partial transection which warrants a surgical exploration in the form of decompression and/or repair. This is done after carrying out appropriate electrophysiological tests such as electroneurography (EnoG) and confirming the occurrence of Wallerian degeneration. An HRCT of the temporal bone would help localize the exact site and extent of the injury and the presence of hematoma, loose bone spicules or fragments, and granulations if any. Facial nerve decompression may be carried out by the middle cranial fossa or transmastoid approach depending on the fracture site. Nerve repair, if required, may be undertaken by end-to-end anastomosis or nerve grafting depending on the extent of nerve loss. Aggressive physiotherapy must continue even after the surgical treatment.

9.1.2 Nose

6. A 25-year-old male complains of watery discharge from his right nostril after being involved in a motor vehicle accident 10 days ago. At that time, he had been hospitalized for a day for a head concussion and minor nosebleed and was not given any medication on discharge. What is to be done for his current complaint?
   (a) Diagnosis
       Cerebrospinal fluid rhinorrhea following head trauma.
       The history of a clear or watery unilateral discharge following trauma to the head is highly suggestive of a cerebrospinal fluid rhinorrhea (CSF). This may be confirmed by asking the patient to bend forward and/or strain, during which the fluid would be seen to escape as droplets which could be collected in a glass bulb. This is also known as the "tea-pot sign." A handkerchief or halo test may also be done to observe if the stain is rimmed by a distinct and darker ring, or if the fabric has a sticky feel, which on drying becomes taut due to the presence of mucus. The history of even a minor nosebleed should not be dismissed. A shearing injury to the nasal mucosa following a blunt head trauma is possible. Head concussion may cause nothing but a mild uneasiness and confirmed by a normal brain CT scan, requiring at the most a day's admission for the purpose of observation in many healthcare centers. The nosebleed is short and transient, may consist of only a few drops of blood at the time of impact, and is explained by the rich vascular supply of the nose.
       However, the roof of the nose, which consists of the cribriform plate of the ethmoid bone, is extremely thin and may be especially vulnerable to a shearing force in case of certain anatomical variations such as a deep olfactory fossa characterized by the type 2 or 3 of the Keros classification. This could result in a fracture of the cribriform plate which might be small in the majority of cases but nonetheless fails to close spontaneously as in cases

where the defect is larger or some congenital anomaly further increases the susceptibility, or other local factors like infection or inflammation are present. In most cases, therefore, the bleeding is extremely short lived, CSF rhinorrhea absent or undetectable, and no complications ensue.

(b) Investigations

A plain coronal paranasal sinus CT combined with a T2-weighted MRI would be the ideal imaging modality to pick up both the bony defect and the presence of a CSF leak without being invasive. Biochemical assessment of the fluid for beta-2 transferrin is more sensitive than for beta-trace protein (BTP) assay, but both are not widely available nor considered to be of much clinical use beyond establishing the fact that the fluid is indeed CSF. A CT-metrizamide scan was the imaging modality used in the pre-MRI era, and fluorescein angiography may be employed on table but are redundant in the current scenario where CT and MRI have been done preoperatively. The leak(s) may be easily seen during surgery or may be elicited by an anesthetic Valsalva procedure. Other routine lab tests may be done.

(c) Treatment

Endoscopic CSF leak closure. This is described in detail in the main chapter.

7. A 10-year-old child hurts his nose while playing with his sibling. There is minimal nosebleed but a large contusion over the nose and also over his left arm. The parents scold the children and tell them to behave, and all is forgotten till the neighbor comes in the next day and advises the family to see a doctor. How would you go about evaluating this patient?

(a) Diagnosis

Trauma to nose with nasal bone fracture.

Children frequently injure their nose while engaging in play. This child too must have suffered a punch to his face from the older child, and the nose being prominent gets injured easily. Being highly vascular as well, nosebleed is common in such injuries. The fact that this child did not suffer a major nosebleed suggests that the impact was minimal. At the same time, a large contusion occurred over the nose and also over the left arm probably because he was trying to ward off the blow.

(b) Investigations

Can this situation be left on its own? Perhaps yes, but certain things need to be looked into. First, the contusions might be the first sign of a bleeding disorder, and a careful family history must be obtained. A full coagulation profile must also be undertaken.

Second, the nose must be carefully examined to rule out a septal hematoma which is very common in such injuries especially in children. A hematoma, if present, needs urgent intervention as described in the main chapter.

Third, children commonly suffer greenstick fractures of the nasal skeleton, which can cause deformity of the nose. After the edema and ecchymosis settle, a clinical examination and an X-ray of the nasal bones would confirm this.

(c) Treatment

If a bleeding disorder and septal hematoma have been ruled out, and a greenstick fracture confirmed, a manual reduction with splinting may be done under general anesthesia, and appropriate symptomatic relief can be given.

Over a period of time as the child is growing, it is possible for the nasal septum to be deviated and the child to complain of nasal obstruction, but this is not a general rule. Treatment is such cases must be given on the particular complaints and needs of the patient.

8. A 35-year-old gentleman riding a motorbike is severely injured and found on the roadside. He is not wearing a helmet but seems to be conscious and alert. He says he was hit from behind by a car which did not stop to help, and that he was thrown off the bike and landed on the grassy kerb. However, there are major injuries over the face, and he is intermittently bleeding from the nose and mouth. He also complains of hip pain and inability to move the left leg. How is this patient to be helped?

(a) Diagnosis

Trauma to face with a Le Fort 2 fracture, fracture/dislocation of left hip, no head injury.

The impact in this case is moderate, and it is a hit and run, so only the account given by the patient is available and cannot be corroborated.

The fact that he was thrown off suggests that he would have landed on his face or on his side, so he has been spared from a true head injury and has not lost consciousness. The sidewalk being grassy also softened the impact. Still, the nose and midface are liable to be hurt considerably by the fall, and there is also the probability of a hip fracture or dislocation.

A Le Fort facial fracture can be easily diagnosed clinically by inserting two fingers into the oral cavity. However, universal precautions and a thorough evaluation are necessary so it is vital to transfer the patient to a hospital as soon as possible. First aid may be given by asking the patient to intermittently pinch his own nose as tightly as possible until the bleeding stops or is lessened. A primary survey to rule out cervical spine injury must be done at the site and an appropriate transfer carried out.

(b) Investigations

X-rays are hardly of any value in such cases. A thorough clinical examination must be carried out to determine what kind of imaging would be required. A plain CT scan of the brain with axial cuts and coronal cuts of the paranasal sinuses can be supplemented with a 3D reformatting to clearly delineate the lines of injury and extent of displacements. Long limb screening with X-rays may also be done with specific views asked for in the event a fracture or dislocation has been found anywhere.

Appropriate laboratory tests are done to rule out medical comorbidities and ensure that the patient is fit for surgical intervention, if any.

Thus, this kind of injury requires a multidisciplinary management with close cooperation between the emergency or trauma surgeon, otolaryngologist, orthopedic surgeon, and also a plastic and reconstructive or maxillofacial surgeon.

(c) Treatment

The epistaxis, if not controlled by the time the patient reaches the hospital, may be tackled by anterior nasal packing with ribbon gauze or, preferably, Merocel. Persistent bleeding may even necessitate a posterior nasal packing. Some centers, however, prefer to perform an endoscopic evaluation of the bleeding site and an endoscopic SPA (sphenopalatine artery) ligation or even angiography and embolization.

The facial fractures may be fixed by wiring and plating. This has been explained in the main chapter.

Other injuries are tackled by the multidisciplinary team.

9. A 60-year-old gentleman undergoes an endoscopic sinus surgery procedure for chronic rhinosinusitis with nasal polyposis. This is the second such surgery for this patient. The following day, severe proptosis is seen over the right eye with limitation of eye movement. What needs to be done for this patient?

(a) Diagnosis

Revision FESS with injury to the anterior ethmoidal artery.

Iatrogenic injury in FESS (functional endoscopic sinus surgery) is a real possibility in cases of revision surgery because the usual landmarks are distorted. Unless extreme caution is exercised, complications such as avulsion of the anterior ethmoidal artery and penetration of the anterior cranial fossa may occur, apart from optic nerve or internal carotid artery injury.

Injury to the anterior ethmoidal artery may not be evident on table or may manifest with just slight bleeding intraoperatively, because the avulsed vessel quickly gets retracted into the orbit. This happens when proper identification of the vessel has not been done. After the surgeon has finished the case, the assistant or resident may not really look out for or notice the slight proptosis that already might have occurred, especially if an SOP (standard operating protocol) does not exist and the chief surgeon has left the theater.

Discovering it several hours later or on the following day is potentially incriminating for the doctor. First, the fact that an iatrogenic injury has occurred even though such a complication is well known. Second, that it was not picked up on time. Third, and in the unfortunate event that blindness has ensued, because it might be too late for a decompression procedure at this stage.

(b) Investigations

An urgent evaluation by both otolaryngologist and ophthalmologist is called for. The vision must be determined by finger perception, finger counting, and reaction of the pupil(s) to light. If there is severe restriction of eye movement, a CT scan of the paranasal sinuses and orbit must be done to rule out a trap-door injury of the floor and medial wall of the orbit, entrapping the inferior rectus or oblique muscle and the medial rectus, respectively.

(c) Treatment

The patient must be returned to theater immediately and a lateral canthotomy done to relieve the tension in the orbit. An endoscopic evaluation may be done to look out for obvious bleeding points, but this is rarely of any use. Cold compresses must be given over the eye in an attempt to reduce the swelling. Antibiotics, anti-inflammatory, and analgesic medications must be given as necessary. The vision must be reviewed periodically, but there is every likelihood that permanent and irreversible blindness has already occurred. The surgeon must brace for the possible malpractice litigation!

9.1.3 Throat

10. A 30-year-old woman was brought to A&E in an unconscious state after a suicidal attempt. A ligature mark is found over her neck and the GCS is 9/15. No other injuries are evident. How would you proceed to deal with her?

(a) Diagnosis

Unconsciousness following partial hanging.

The young lady in this case attempted to take her own life but did not succeed. Probably she was desperate but still hoped to be rescued. Partial hanging occurred because a support was present under the feet to prevent complete suspension of the body. Such victims/survivors fortunately do not know the nitty-gritty of how to successfully hang themselves, but black humor aside, there may be a serious but subconscious motivation to live.

The ligature used in such cases is usually a long but thin cloth such as a bed sheet or an item of clothing. A rope might not be used in many cases. Thus, tightening of the knot of the ligature is just enough to shut off the blood supply to the brain, resulting in anoxia and unconsciousness. The body is then suspended partially until a timely rescue takes place. This could be variable, and the resultant condition of the patient depends on the amount of time the patient has been unconscious.

Lack of any other injury marks on the neck or elsewhere on the body helps to rule out foul play such as strangulation or assault, but a careful search must be made for the same.

(b) Investigations

A CT scan brain would confirm the extent of intracranial injury. X-rays of the cervical spine may be taken to rule out a fracture. The otolaryngologist may find indirect evidence of venous congestion in the neck and head due to the (partial) hanging in the form of petechial hemorrhages over the tympanic membrane(s). Whenever possible, the larynx must be visualized by fiber optic laryngoscopy to rule out mucosal injury.

Routine laboratory investigations are also carried out.

(c) Treatment

Prompt treatment is directed toward reversing any kind of anoxic brain injury. A GCS of 9/15 may be managed without endotracheal intubation, but vigilance must be maintained for the occurrence of stridor. Brain edema must be treated with appropriate medications such as mannitol and steroids. Supportive and symptomatic treatment must be given. A thorough ENT evaluation and review must be carried out, but generally no active intervention is required. All the changes taking place are usually due to venous congestion and would settle over a period of time. Hyoid fracture is usually seen in strangulation and not hanging and does not require any major intervention.

11. A 20-year-old farmer is rushed to A&E after consuming insecticide. He is semi-conscious and frothing at the mouth. The GCS is 10/15, and there is stridor and signs of respiratory distress. What is to be done for this patient?

(a) Diagnosis

Airway and neurotoxic injury due to consumption of organophosphorus compound.

Farmers, especially in the third world, are highly susceptible to injury with insecticides or pesticides: first, because of intentional self-harm and attempt of suicide; second, due to chronic and occupational exposure; and third, due to accidental ingestion owing to inattention, illiteracy, ignorance, intoxication, or poor illumination where such chemicals are stored.

Such compounds are poisonous to the body by virtue of their ability to interfere with cellular function, especially the function of nerve organs and endocrine organs. They are also directly toxic to the skin and mucosa, causing severe congestion and inflammation at such sites. Acute ARDS (adult respiratory distress syndrome) may occur due to cessation of gas exchange in the lungs following central brain injury and diaphragmatic paralysis. Unconsciousness soon follows, and the condition is potentially fatal if not treated in time. The frothing at the mouth and respiratory distress is highly suggestive of ARDS.

(b) Investigations

A detailed laboratory and toxicological evaluation must be done expediently and the patient managed in a critical care setting with good infrastructure such as the availability of ventilators. Chest X-rays are required to confirm and determine the lung injury resulting from ARDS. Other investigations may be required on a case to case basis.

(c) Treatment

Even though the GCS is not so poor, an endotracheal intubation must be done right away to not only bypass a swollen, inflamed airway with risk of asphyxiation, but also because the ARDS is usually progressive and may kill the patient. The ARDS and metabolic or neurological injury must be tackled by the emergency and intensive care teams. An endotracheal intubation may not always be possible because of airway narrowing. In such cases, an emergency tracheotomy must be done. Depending on the severity of poisoning, an elective tracheotomy may follow the intubation so that the upper airway inflammation has had time to settle. Details of this are given in the main chapter.

The patient must be kept on long-term surveillance to prevent airway stenosis either following the poisoning or the intubation. Psychiatric consultation and counseling may be required for cases of attempted suicide. Socioeconomic aspects need to be looked into such as the easy availability of toxic substances and accidental poisoning.

12. A 40-year-old male is brought to A&E with his head, face, and upper torso covered in blood. He is unconscious with a GCS of 6/15. How is this patient to be treated?

   (a) Diagnosis

   Hemorrhagic shock due to assault to neck.

   Though it is difficult to determine the site of injury at this stage, it would be safe to assume that it is the neck since all the major vessels are encountered here, thus explaining the massive blood loss and shock due to exsanguination. The pulse and blood pressure would therefore be very low, leading to hypoxia or anoxia to the brain and the unconscious state. So the primary survey would suggest the above diagnosis.

   (b) Investigations

   In such a case, investigations would have to wait till the patient has been resuscitated. The ABCs of shock would have to be looked into first. Thus, the airway must be established right away. This may be done with endotracheal intubation but could be extremely difficult in such a situation. A tracheotomy would be ideal but again may prove difficult and time consuming. Assuming that a cut throat injury has occurred, it might be that some kind of airway already exists and is allowing the patient to maintain a minimal respiration.

   Therefore, the patient must be expediently revived from the state of shock by the institution of an intravenous access and rushing fluids. As soon as the pulse and blood pressure have been somewhat improved, access to the airway must be ensured by either intubation or tracheotomy, though the latter would be preferable to a blind intubation because of the severely distorted neck anatomy.

   A quick secondary survey must be done to rule out other injuries, and the patient must be taken up for definitive neck exploration in the operation room.

   Investigations other than routine laboratory tests are not required at this point. If there is no active bleeding from the wound and the patient is stabilized, a CT scan may be arranged as quickly as possible to determine the nature and extent of deeper injury. In the case of active bleeding, a CT angiography or Doppler may have to be done expediently to determine the site of the bleed.

   (c) Treatment

   Exploration of the wound is paramount. It would also reveal the exact nature of the injury and also confirm that there has been a penetrating neck trauma. The neck wound management should proceed as explained in the main chapter.

13. A 3-year-old child has been crying continuously, refusing feeds, and drooling from the mouth for a few hours. He is brought to the hospital by his mother who reports that he was playing with a remote-controlled toy car while at home.

There is no evidence of respiratory distress in the patient, but he is lying limp and listless in his mother's lap. What do you wish to do for the patient?

(a) Diagnosis

Ingestion/inhalation of foreign body.

Foreign body ingestion or aspiration (inhalation) is extremely common in this age group, and normally toys and gadgets with batteries and removable parts should never be given to small children to play with. It is possible that the child has put a small part or battery of the toy car into his mouth, and this has either entered the airway or the esophagus of the baby.

A battery causes severe inflammation of the mucosa, which could involve the airway even if the foreign body has entered the digestive tract. The drooling and refusal of feeds are explained by this and also the crankiness and incessant crying. There is also the possibility of it being in the airway but not occluding the lumen completely. The initial choking or cough may have gone unnoticed, and the child may be already fatigued by the respiratory distress and is therefore listless. This is a sign of grave danger.

(b) Investigations

A plain X-ray neck and chest in both lateral and anteroposterior views must be taken to confirm the presence of the foreign body and the status of the lungs.

Routine laboratory investigations are usually not required as this is a dire emergency.

(c) Treatment

Emergency bronchoscopy/esophagoscopy must be performed under anesthesia in the operation room. Details of this are given in the main chapter.

14. A 50-year-old lady presents to the outpatient department with hoarseness of voice and dyspnea on exertion. She had suffered a stroke 6 months ago and had been hospitalized and treated in intensive care for a month. She has now recovered fully except for the above complaints. What do you think the patient is suffering from?

(a) Diagnosis

Vocal cord paralysis/granuloma with subglottic stenosis.

Patients with stroke may need to be intubated and managed in critical care. An otolaryngologist is usually not called in except for evaluation of a complaint of dysphagia, if any. Upon recovery and discharge of the patient, otolaryngological follow-up is thus never done unless the patient has a particular complaint.

Vocal cord injury due to endotracheal intubation is more common than usually believed. The cord may get dislocated, or a granuloma may develop at the site of mucosal injury. Stenosis is common at the site of the endotracheal tube cuff due to increased pressure and lack of adequate deflation.

(b) Investigations

Plain X-ray chest, CT scan, or MRI would confirm the diagnosis. A laryngoscopy would also reveal the same. Routine investigations must be done as a surgical procedure might be necessary.

(c) Treatment
Treatment of vocal cord paralysis/granuloma or stenosis is given in the main chapter. Malpractice litigation is unusual in such cases as no guidelines or SOPs exist for this very common complication.

9.1.4 Miscellaneous

15. A 50-year-old lady presents to the clinic complaining of inability to close the mouth. She reveals that it happened while yawning and has occurred several times in the past.
    (a) Diagnosis
        Recurrent dislocation/subluxation of the mandible.
        The temporomandibular joint (TMJ) is prone to dislocation or subluxation, which is common in both males and females irrespective of age, though it might be said that middle aged or elderly females are more susceptible. This is because of less muscular strength and gradual effacement of the temporomandibular joint because of increasing age and loss of dentition. The history of recurring episodes is thus common in such patients, and the most common trigger is a forceful or deep yawn.
        Anterior dislocation is more common because the glenoid fossa is shallower anteriorly. Both the joints may be involved. This causes stretching of the lateral pterygoid muscles thus locking the mouth in the open position.
    (b) Investigations
        Suspected cases must be investigated for connective tissue disorders. Routine laboratory investigations are necessary because surgical therapy may have to be undertaken in the event of recurrent dislocation.
    (c) Treatment
    Usually the mandible gets dislocated anteriorly and may easily be reduced by bilateral and symmetrical manual pressure in a downward direction just behind the last molar tooth.
    A barrel bandage must be given to prevent immediate recurrence which is common in these cases as the joint is lax.
    Definitive surgery may have to be planned electively. Details are given in the main chapter.

Conclusion

Trauma, one must understand, affects an otherwise normal person or one already having an ailment and must therefore be managed in the appropriate context. Basic facts in the anatomy and pathophysiology of head and neck trauma must be at ready disposal in order to optimize trauma management in this region.

Quiz

1. Intracellular movement of sodium following arterial occlusion occurs within:
   - (a) 10 seconds
   - (b) 10 minutes
   - (c) 10 hours
   - (d) 10 days
2. Zone 3 of perfusion refers to the:
   - (a) Cell and its membranes
   - (b) Interstitial space
   - (c) Cardiopulmonary system
   - (d) Capillary circulation
3. In human beings, the skin is supplied by:
   - (a) Septocutaneous arteries
   - (b) Direct cutaneous arteries
   - (c) Musculocutaneous arteries
   - (d) Fasciocutaneous arteries
4. The maximum length of flap undermining to reduce wound tension is:
   - (a) 2 cm
   - (b) 3 cm
   - (c) 4 cm
   - (d) 5 cm
5. All are implicated in reperfusion injury except:
   - (a) Low cardiac output
   - (b) Lactic acidosis (hyperosmosis)
   - (c) Polymorphonuclear cells (neutrophils)
   - (d) Xanthine oxidase/superoxide dismutase
6. The most influential factor in improving the viability of a flap is:
   - (a) Vasodilators
   - (b) Flap delay
   - (c) Metabolic manipulation
   - (d) Rheology

© Springer Nature Singapore Pte Ltd. 2018
J. Das, *Trauma in Otolaryngology*, https://doi.org/10.1007/978-981-10-6361-9

7. The advantages offered by a flap delay may last up to:
   (a) 2 weeks
   (b) 4 weeks
   (c) 6 weeks
   (d) 8 weeks
8. Flap delay is successful due to all the following except:
   (a) Closing of arteriovenous shunts
   (b) Improvement in blood flow
   (c) Conditioning of flap to ischemia
   (d) Reduction in cellular immunity
9. All the three forms of NOS (nitric oxide synthase) can be expressed by:
   (a) Macrophages
   (b) Keratinocytes
   (c) Langerhans cells
   (d) Fibroblasts
10. The normal skin ratio of type 1 to type 3 collagen is:
    (a) 3:1
    (b) 4:1
    (c) 5:1
    (d) 2:1
11. Which of the following is not a hair-bearing part of the nasal lining?
    (a) Nasal facets
    (b) Membranous septum
    (c) Nasal alae
    (d) Vestibule
12. The longest (most delayed) recorded complication of a frontal sinus fracture is:
    (a) 10 years
    (b) 15 years
    (c) 25 years
    (d) 30 years
13. Foreign bodies in the upper aerodigestive tract are best delineated by a:
    (a) X-ray neck
    (b) USG neck
    (c) CT scan
    (d) MRI scan
14. The maximum length of a free osteocutaneous flap is obtained from the:
    (a) Iliac crest
    (b) Fibula
    (c) Radius
    (d) Rib
15. Facial paralysis may occur in transverse temporal bone fractures as often as:
    (a) 25%
    (b) 50%
    (c) 75%
    (d) 100%

16. The facial function that is the last one to recover from facial nerve palsy is:
    (a) Eye closure
    (b) Ballooning of cheek
    (c) Wide smile
    (d) Facial symmetry

17. Evoked electromyography is also known as:
    (a) NET
    (b) MST
    (c) ENoG
    (d) EMG

18. All the following are caused by some form of trauma except:
    (a) Cauliflower ear
    (b) Swimmer's ear
    (c) Lop ear
    (d) Frostbite

19. Teapot sign may be seen in:
    (a) Traumatic epistaxis
    (b) CSF leak
    (c) Orbital complication of FESS
    (d) Complication of Caldwell-Luc procedure

20. Battle's sign is another name for:
    (a) Mastoid contusion
    (b) Raccoon eyes
    (c) Traumatic facial palsy
    (d) Naso-orbito-ethmoid fracture

21. Penetrating injury of the head, face, and neck is most life-threatening in:
    (a) Zone 1
    (b) Zone 2
    (c) Zone 3
    (d) All of the above

22. Fracture of the hyoid as seen in hanging is best treated by:
    (a) Closed reduction
    (b) Open reduction
    (c) Open reduction with fixation
    (d) Conservative management

23. Craniofacial disjunction may be found in:
    (a) Le Fort 2 fracture
    (b) Le Fort 3 fracture
    (c) Dentoalveolar fracture
    (d) Mandibular fracture

24. Radiation exposure is measured in:
    (a) Centigray
    (b) Gray
    (c) Millisievert
    (d) Sievert

25. Correction for hypoglobus is required if the displacement of the globe exceeds:
    (a) 3 mm
    (b) 4 mm
    (c) 5 mm
    (d) 6 mm
26. The primary component of a facial transplant is the:
    (a) Vascular pedicle
    (b) Neuroangiosome
    (c) Neural plasticity
    (d) Cutaneous dermatome
27. The mandible most commonly fractures at the:
    (a) Ramus
    (b) Symphysis
    (c) Condyle
    (d) Body
28. Massive hemothorax is defined as the collection of blood in a hemithorax that exceeds:
    (a) 1000 mL
    (b) 1500 mL
    (c) 2000 mL
    (d) 2500 mL
29. In the ATLS protocol, the first step is:
    (a) Resuscitation
    (b) Primary survey
    (c) Secondary survey
    (d) Definitive care
30. All are examples of blunt injuries except:
    (a) Rotational
    (b) Stretch and tear
    (c) Barotrauma
    (d) Deceleration

Answers to the above quiz are provided herewith.

1. (b)
2. (b)
3. (c)
4. (c)
5. (a)
6. (b)
7. (c)
8. (d)
9. (b)
10. (b)
11. (b)
12. (c)
13. (c)
14. (b)
15. (b)
16. (c)
17. (c)
18. (c)
19. (b)
20. (a)
21. (b)
22. (d)
23. (b)
24. (c)
25. (a)
26. (b)
27. (c)
28. (b)
29. (b)
30. (c)